T0260564

The Elite Facial Surgery Practice

Development and Management

E. Gaylon McCollough, MD, FACS
Founder and Chief Operational Officer
McCollough Plastic Surgery Clinic
The McCollough Institute for Appearance & Health
Gulf Shores, Alabama, USA

35 illustrations

Thieme
New York · Stuttgart · Delhi · Rio de Janeiro

Executive Editor: Timothy Hiscock
Managing Editor: Elizabeth Palumbo
Director, Editorial Services: Mary Jo Casey
Production Editor: Torsten Scheihagen
International Production Director: Andreas Schabert
Editorial Director: Sue Hodgson
International Marketing Director: Fiona Henderson
International Sales Director: Louisa Turrell
Director of Institutional Sales: Adam Bernacki
Senior Vice President and Chief Operating Officer:
    Sarah Vanderbilt
President: Brian D. Scanlan
Cover art: Stedmann B. McCollough and McCollough
    Architecture, Gulf Shores, AL
Illustrator: Daniela de Castro
Printer: King Printing

Library of Congress Cataloging-in-Publication Data
Names: McCollough, E. Gaylon.
Title: The elite facial surgery practice : development and
    management / E. Gaylon McCollough, MD, FACS,
    Founder and Chief Operational Officer, McCollough
    Plastic Surgery Clinic, The McCollough Institute for
    Appearance & Health, Gulf Shores, Alabama, USA.
Description: New York : Thieme, [2017]
Identifiers: LCCN 2017027743| ISBN 9781626236448
    (print) | ISBN 9781626236455 (e-book)
Subjects: LCSH: Face--Surgery. | Surgery, Plastic.
Classification: LCC RD119.5.F33 M33
2017 | DDC 617.5/2059--dc23 LC record available at
https://lccn.loc.gov/2017027743

Important note: Medicine is an ever-changing science undergoing continual development. Research and clinical experience are continually expanding our knowledge, in particular our knowledge of proper treatment and drug therapy. Insofar as this book mentions any dosage or application, readers may rest assured that the authors, editors, and publishers have made every effort to ensure that such references are in accordance with **the state of knowledge at the time of production of the book**.

Nevertheless, this does not involve, imply, or express any guarantee or responsibility on the part of the publishers in respect to any dosage instructions and forms of applications stated in the book. **Every user is requested to examine carefully** the manufacturers' leaflets accompanying each drug and to check, if necessary in consultation with a physician or specialist, whether the dosage schedules mentioned therein or the contraindications stated by the manufacturers differ from the statements made in the present book. Such examination is particularly important with drugs that are either rarely used or have been newly released on the market. Every dosage schedule or every form of application used is entirely at the user's own risk and responsibility. The authors and publishers request every user to report to the publishers any discrepancies or inaccuracies noticed. If errors in this work are found after publication, errata will be posted at www.thieme.com on the product description page.

Some of the product names, patents, and registered designs referred to in this book are in fact registered trademarks or proprietary names even though specific reference to this fact is not always made in the text. Therefore, the appearance of a name without designation as proprietary is not to be construed as a representation by the publisher that it is in the public domain.

Copyright © 2018 by Thieme Medical Publishers, Inc.

Thieme Publishers New York
333 Seventh Avenue, New York, NY 10001 USA
+1 800 782 3488, customerservice@thieme.com

Thieme Publishers Stuttgart
Rüdigerstrasse 14, 70469 Stuttgart, Germany
+49 [0]711 8931 421, customerservice@thieme.de

Thieme Publishers Delhi
A-12, Second Floor, Sector-2, Noida-201301
Uttar Pradesh, India
+91 120 45 566 00, customerservice@thieme.in

Thieme Publishers Rio de Janeiro, Thieme Publicações Ltda.
Edifício Rodolpho de Paoli, 25° andar
Av. Nilo Peçanha, 50 – Sala 2508,
Rio de Janeiro 20020-906 Brasil
+55 21 3172-2297 / +55 21 3172-1896

Cover design: Thieme Publishing Group
Typesetting by DiTech Process Solutions

Printed in the United States of America by King Printing
5 4 3 2 1

ISBN 978-1-62623-644-8

Also available as an e-book:
eISBN 978-1-62623-645-5

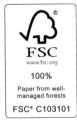

FSC
www.fsc.org
100%
Paper from well-managed forests
FSC® C103101

"Elite: the part of a group regarded as the. . .
most distinguished."

—*Webster's New World College Dictionary, Third Edition, Simon & Schuster, 1998*

Contents

Preface

An elite facial surgery practice depends upon mastering not only the surgical, psychological, and interpersonal skills required, but also those of a business nature—economic, managerial, and legal.

In mentoring the next generation of appearance-enhancing surgeons I call upon more than 40 years of experience. I guide readers through the process of obtaining the best training and continuing education possible, creating an environment conducive to elective surgery, establishing lasting doctor–patient relationships, and efficiently managing a solo practice, clinic, or institutional department.

In contrast to classical textbook offerings, this publication does not dwell on how facial surgery procedures are performed, but rather on when—and upon whom—they are indicated. I focus on how to win the confidence of patients and create an environment that delivers an extraordinary level of care. Specific techniques, materials, and products employed by me in my practice are detailed in textbooks, peer-reviewed journals, and presentations during conferences. In this book you will find trade secrets that will help you create lasting doctor–patient relationships, conduct personalized postoperative care, deal with unfortunate outcomes, manage dissatisfied patients, minimize risks of legal proceedings, and defend yourself in court.

Facial surgeons who adhere to the practices and principles herein offered will be better prepared to face—with confidence—whatever challenges lie ahead. They will have a competitive edge in a faction of the personal-enhancement industry that rewards extraordinary service, and the lifestyle thereunto aligned.

E. Gaylon McCollough, MD, FACS
Past President:
American Academy of Facial Plastic and Reconstructive Surgery,
American Board of Facial Plastic and Reconstructive Surgery,
American Academy of Facial Plastic and Reconstructive Surgery Foundation
Fellowship Director,
American Academy of Facial Plastic and Reconstructive Surgery

Acknowledgments

I wish to credit my facial plastic surgery fellowship mentors Drs. Jack R. Anderson, Richard C. Webster, and Walter E. Berman for sharing their own practice protocols with me. From their examples—coupled with my own experiences—the practice model herein offered took shape.

I also wish to credit two other mentors. Dr. James J. Hicks was chairman of the Division of Otolaryngology at UAB Medical Center in Birmingham, Alabama, when I was a resident in the early 1970s. Dr. Hicks was also managing partner of one of the largest private otolaryngology/head and neck surgery practices in history. I would be remiss if I didn't give credit to Coach Paul "Bear" Bryant, under whose tutelage I studied and played to a national championship season in the early 1960s. His assessment and motivational skills were unparalleled during his time.

Each of the men referenced above was an insightful instructor and motivator. Each was eager to share his expertise in building successful surgical practices, postgraduate educational curricula, and (in Coach Bryant's case) an athletic program that football coaches have, ever since, attempted to emulate.

It is my hope that this book will also prove beneficial to fellowship directors and residency program chairmen as they prepare aspiring young facial surgeons for the road ahead.

Author's Note

On the Shoulders of Giants

In a classic Greek epic (*The Civil War*) two armies were poised on either side of a hill, ready to meet in battle. From their positions on the ground, neither army could see the exact position or size of the other. Military general Didacus Stella turned to a lieutenant and ordered, "Lift the dwarfs on the shoulders of the giants. From that elevated position, the dwarfs can see more than the giants."

In like manner, each generation of physicians is able to see and understand more than previous generations, not because of the greatness of the current generation's size or the keenness of its eyes, but because it rests upon the foundations built by predecessors. This premise provided the inspiration that (in the 1980s) led me to write *Shoulders of Giants.*[1] It was a tribute to my mentors and to the giants who preceded them.

A decade afterward, I wrote *Before and After: Proof that the Past Is Prologue.*[2] It, too, is based upon a venerable axiom—one handed down from generation to generation within the Native American community: "To understand the present and see into the future, study the past." Simply stated, human behavior is destined to repeat. And, only a few heed the admonitions of past masters. These are the members of each generation who avoid repeating avoidable mistakes.

I often recall the advice offered by my father. "You can learn life's lessons by one of two methods: by trial and error, or by heeding the advice of knowledgeable people." With that thought in mind, let us reflect upon the wisdom and admonitions offered by the profession's founding fathers.

The following is a contemporary translation[3] (from the original Greek) of an oath credited to Hippocrates, the "Father of Medicine." It is the basis upon which every thought, every urging, every recommendation offered in this book is based. The Hippocratic Oath is a reminder that we are, first, physicians, then facial surgeons, a remembrance that every patient and member of a physician's staff must recognize, by our actions.

Although the majority of doctors were asked to swear allegiance to "the Oath" upon graduating from medical school, we may not have realized the far-reaching implications of its words.

It matters that I publish a copy of the Oath at the beginning of this book, and recommend each reader pay close attention to the document's written— and implied—admonitions. The second and third bullet points have particular significance in the message herein presented.

- I swear to fulfill, to the best of my ability and judgment, this covenant:
- I will respect the hard-won scientific gains of those physicians in whose steps I walk, and gladly share such knowledge as is mine with those who are to follow.
- I will apply, for the benefit of the sick, all measures [that] are required, avoiding those twin traps of overtreatment and therapeutic nihilism.
- I will remember that there is art to medicine as well as science, and that warmth, sympathy, and understanding may outweigh the surgeon's knife or the chemist's drug.

- I will not be ashamed to say "I know not," nor will I fail to call in my colleagues when the skills of another are needed for a patient's recovery.
- I will respect the privacy of my patients, for their problems are not disclosed to me that the world may know. Most especially I must tread with care in matters of life and death. If it is given me to save a life, all thanks. But it may also be within my power to take a life; this awesome responsibility must be faced with great humbleness and awareness of my own frailty. Above all, I must not play at God.
- I will remember that I do not treat a fever chart, a cancerous growth, but a sick human being, whose illness may affect the person's family and economic stability. My responsibility includes these related problems, if I am to care adequately for the sick.
- I will prevent disease whenever I can, for prevention is preferable to cure.
- I will remember that I remain a member of society, with special obligations to all my fellow human beings, those [who are] sound of mind and body as well as the infirm.
- If I do not violate this oath, may I enjoy life and art, respected while I live and remembered with affection thereafter. May I always act so as to preserve the finest traditions of my calling and may I long experience the joy of healing those who seek my help.

Twenty centuries later, another "giant," Dr. Tinsley R. Harrison, wrote the following in the introduction of the medical textbook that still carries his name.

"No greater calling can befall a human being than to be called a physician. In the care of the suffering he needs technical skill, scientific knowledge, and human understanding. He who uses these with courage, with humility, and with wisdom, will provide a unique service for his fellowman and will build an enduring edifice of character within himself. The physician should ask of his destiny no more than this; he should be content with no less."[4]

I knew Dr. Harrison. For an entire summer during medical school, he was one of my mentors. His words and admonitions embodied those of Hippocrates. They underlie my intent to "share such knowledge as is mine with those who are to follow."

The principles and protocols herein shared are constructed from building blocks I learned from "knowledgeable people" (giants who established and maintained elite practices). I also include a healthy mix of "trial and error" experiences.

1. Shoulders of Giants, McCollough, E.G., Albright Publishing, 1986
2. Before and After, McCollough, E.G., Compass Press, 1994
3. Written in 1964 by Louis Lasagna, Academic Dean of the School of Medicine at Tufts University, and used in many medical schools today.
4. Harrison's Principles of Internal Medicine, Kasper, D., Fauci, F., Longo, D., et al. 19th ed. McGraw Hill Education, 2015.

Prudence in Preparation

1 Academic Pathways to a Practice in Facial Surgery

No one-size-fits-all model exists to become a facial surgeon. However, common characteristics can be found among the most successful of the lot: an eye for beauty and harmony, good interpersonal skills, and attention to detail.

Five primary educational pathways provide the prerequisite training needed to develop a practice composed of a high volume of aesthetic facial surgery:

1. Otolaryngology–head and neck Surgery, coupled with a postresidency fellowship in facial plastic and reconstructive surgery.
2. Plastic surgery, with prerequisite residency training in general surgery, otolaryngology–head and neck surgery, orthopaedic surgery, or urological surgery. A postresidency fellowship in facial plastic and reconstructive surgery is helpful, if the plastic surgery residency program did not include a high volume of aesthetic facial surgery.
3. Ophthalmology, with a postresidency fellowship in oculoplastic surgery.
4. Dermatology, with a postresidency fellowship in procedural dermatology or Mohs's surgery.
5. Oral and maxillofacial surgery (OMFS) with a postresidency fellowship in cosmetic surgery of the face, head, and neck.

Each of the preceding routes has advantages—and disadvantages—compared with the others. It is not the purpose of this book to recommend one over the other. Aspiring facial surgeons should explore each route and determine in their own mind which best fits the scope of practice to which they aspire.

Not all practices devoted to aesthetic and reconstructive facial surgery are alike, nor should they be. Even in limiting one's practice to aesthetic and reconstructive surgery within the head and neck, it is difficult to be all things to all people, even if one would like to be.

I was once told by an international business consultant that the extraordinary individual or corporation "finds its place in the universe." It fills an existing void, and fills it better than the rest.

I recommend that physicians decide where their interests and skills best apply, and focus on the training model, procedures, and nature of practice that best suit them. For example, there are surgeons who only perform aesthetic rhinoplasty. Others perform functional, reconstructive, and aesthetic rhinoplasty. Still others specialize in total nasal reconstruction using regional flaps and composite grafts.

Aesthetic procedures range from isolated superficial (level I) skin resurfacing to full facial rejuvenation with facelifting, blepharoplasty, and level III skin resurfacing at the same sitting.

Some surgeons specialize in periorbital aesthetic surgery, others in orthognathic procedures that reposition malaligned facial skeletal features.

To become an elite facial surgeon, a physician must explore the pros and cons of the alternatives and be prepared to deal with the consequences thereof.

From a credentialing standpoint, some pathways make it easier to obtain hospital and surgicenter privileges and malpractice coverage to perform certain facial procedures than others. And although it might require additional years of training, one can always change focus or specialties, should one recognize that another pathway best fits one's personal and professional ambitions.

As an aspiring young surgeon I was faced with this same decision as referenced above. I concluded that the most logical course of training for me to specialize in facial surgery was otolaryngology–head and neck surgery.

In this pathway, at least 4 years of postgraduate training are spent in diagnosing and treating conditions within the face, nose, periorbital region, and neck. Many of the procedures that treat traumatic and pathological conditions in these regions of the head and neck are approached using the same, or very similar, incisions and dissection planes as are aesthetic procedures.

This prerequisite training, coupled with a 1-year fellowship in facial plastic and reconstructive surgery (American Academy of Facial Plastic and Reconstructive Surgery [AAFPRS]), provided the training and credentialing I needed to become a facial plastic surgeon.

In the 21st century, board certification is an important indication of a surgeon's prerequisite training. Certification by the American Board of Facial Plastic and Reconstructive Surgery has been deemed "equivalent" to that by American Board of Medical Specialties (ABMS) boards that certify in plastic and reconstructive surgery of the face, nose, head, and neck.

The second most common route to a practice in aesthetic surgery is through a plastic surgery residency. This course of study generally requires at least 3 years of general surgery training or a board-qualified residency in otolaryngology–head and neck surgery, orthopaedic surgery, or urology.

During a residency in plastic surgery the trainee is exposed to facial surgery but must also be prepared to pass an oral and written examination in aesthetic and reconstructive surgery of the breast, body, and hand.

While in today's medical environment the credentialing part of the equation (through the American Board of Plastic Surgery) may be more easily solved, the experience in actually performing and assisting on facial surgery procedures and postoperative management is, in many programs, less intensive than with the otolaryngology–head and neck surgery/AAFPRS fellowship route.

Third on the list is the pathway through ophthalmology, with a postresidency fellowship in oculoplastic surgery. Board-certified ophthalmologists who pursue this route are duly qualified to perform aesthetic and reconstructive surgery in the periorbital region upon entering practice. In recent years, some have also acquired expertise in performing brow and midface lifting procedures.

Oculoplastic surgeons are also called upon to assist surgeons in all of the listed specialties in managing surgical complications, reconstructing traumatic deformities and cancer defects following Mohs's surgery in the periorbital region.

As recently as the 1980s, dermatology was considered a medical specialty. However, with the advent of Mohs's surgery, hair restoration, skin resurfacing technologies, and postresidency fellowships in procedural dermatology, many dermatologists focus on aesthetic and reconstructive procedures within the head and neck region.

Procedural dermatology and Mohs's surgery fellowships provide dermatology residents (and fellows) with advanced training in dealing with patients seeking rejuvenation procedures. An increasing number of board-certified dermatologists are acquiring training in aesthetic/cosmetic procedures.

In the 1960s progressive OMFS residency programs joined with medical schools to provide a doctor of medicine degree, in addition to the doctor of dental surgery (DDS) degree, at the conclusion of an oral surgery residency. This, coupled with the advent of orthognathic surgery, provided opportunities to enter regions of the face beyond the oral cavity, maxilla, and mandible.

Surgeons with OMFS training became involved with the American Academy of Cosmetic Surgery. Many earned board certification by the American Board of Cosmetic Surgery and offer comprehensive facial surgery services.

In short, if one chooses to spend one's professional career performing aesthetic and reconstructive surgery in the face and neck, there are several pathways toward that end. My recommendation is this: examine each of the options herein presented and follow the one that best fits one's own personal and professional goals.

Clearly, training and skill development does not end with residency or fellowships. There is a reason it is called the "practice" of medicine and surgery. Continuing educational programs allow physicians with solid foundational backgrounds to adopt and adapt to new technologies and procedures as their interests evolve.

An eye and appreciation for the arts and sciences of proportion and harmony appears to attract individuals from a wide variety of backgrounds to aesthetic medicine and surgery. The ability to visualize an outcome in one's mind before the operation is initiated gives one a distinct advantage over peers who do not possess such abilities.

Naturally, the dexterity required to perform delicate operations is a necessary skill; but there is more to having a successful facial surgery practice than adeptly cutting, carving, and aligning body parts that anatomically reside above the shoulders.

2 The Golden Rule of Facial Surgery

Dr. Jack Anderson referred to facial surgery as "psychological surgery," in that many of the individuals who seek the advice and services of a facial surgeon carry the burden of hurtful comments that have left deep-seated scars in their psyche. The surgeon's role is to identify the patient's current self-image, then have an open and honest discussion as to how the surgeon and the patient will need to work in concert for the patient to shed the old self-image and replace it with the new.

For most facial surgeons, performance of the surgical procedures is the easy work. Preoperative screening, counseling, and postoperative nurturing required by a patient undergoing appearance-altering surgery is a greater challenge. The harder work is dealing with the business side of the practice. Hopefully, the following chapters of this book will make that part of the practice easier for future generations of surgeons.

Unlike many of our medical colleagues, facial surgeons make patients look and feel worse—temporarily. As caretakers, part of our role is to help them through these challenging times. To do so, facial surgeons must have the patience and temperament required to be nurturers. They must inform patients that healing from surgery is a process (progression) of nature, some of which is simply beyond the surgeon's control, and that the patient also plays an integral role in determining the outcome of the operation and whether the course of recovery will proceed "as per usual."

Patients should be informed in advance about their postoperative appearance and reassured that once swelling and bruising subside, things will improve. It is helpful to provide (with the patients' written consent) photographs of previous patients at various stages of healing. Even so, some patients require more reassurance than others. And facial surgeons and their staff must provide such assurances with compassion and conviction.

Here is where a surgeon's inner character comes into play. Never, ever, lie to a patient! If a problem exists during the postoperative period, admit that the problem exists; then reassure the patient that the two of you must stick together and "work through" the problem. Once lied to, patients will not trust anything else they are told.

I frequently consult with patients who are dissatisfied with the outcomes of surgery performed by other surgeons. Because they were not told the truth, many of these patients lost faith in the medical profession. The first order of business is to rehabilitate the profession. It is not productive to say bad things about previous surgeons. It is best to refrain from joining the patient in deriding other doctors. I have found it helpful to respond to negative comments about colleagues by saying the following: "I was not there at the time of your surgery, or during the healing process. Anything I say would be speculation. We have to deal with the situation as it now exists. Let's see what we can do to try and make it better."

Pay close attention to every word in the sentences above. Let there be no guarantee—stated or implied—that you will make things better. Rather, state that you are going to attempt to do so.

Here's an additional narrative that tends to win the trust of patients. Look them in the eye and say, "Regardless of what may have occurred in the past, I will never lie to you. If, after surgery, I tell you everything is healing as expected, trust me. If I see a problem, you will not have to point it out to me. I will point it out to you. And we will work through it." If repeated with conviction, these words have proven to establish the kind of doctor-patient relationship that serves both parties through good times and bad. As soon as I speak them, I can see a sense of relief come over the patient. The doctor-patient relationship I want to establish has taken a giant leap forward.

This is the initial—and crucial—part of the rehabilitation process. Surgeons must abide by the promise they make to the patient. In like manner, patients must do their part. I will say more on postoperative management later.

The bottom line is simple. And it's 20 centuries old: the Golden Rule. Treat patients in the same manner that you'd like to be treated.

3 The Office and Staff

During interviews with candidates applying for facial surgery fellowships (who, temporarily, become an integral member of the fellowship director's staff), I like to ask if the candidate enjoyed courses in psychology and clinical rotations in psychiatry. If candidates indicate that they did not enjoy those courses of study, I suggest that a career in facial surgery may not be their best choice, certainly not one that focuses on elective aesthetic surgery.

The most successful facial surgeons I know enjoy the nurturing part of the care they provide. They genuinely enjoy personal interaction with the patients and work toward establishing long-term, professional relationships with the families and friends of patients. On more occasions than one might imagine, a family or friend comes with a patient for a single purpose: to size up the surgeon. Nurturing the patient's circle of supporters often translates to one or more of them scheduling surgery.

Here I pause to share another teaching point, one that I emphasize the first day a new fellow is "on the job." Just before the fellow and I go into the consultation room to see a new patient, I turn to the fellow and ask, "Why are we going in to see this patient? What is our primary objective?"

In one way or another, most fellows answer, "To schedule the patient for a procedure." This is my opportunity to imbue an indelible mark into the mind of the aspiring facial surgeon. I answer, "The correct answer is to establish a relationship of mutual trust. Once such a relationship is solidified, the patient will trust my recommendations and generally go forward with what is recommended, today and for decades to come." I will provide more on the art of the consultation with patients seeking to enhance their appearance later.

The doctor's expanded office staff will serve as an asset, or a liability. Among all challenges, this might be the practice enhancement factor that is given the least attention by a physician.

On a return flight from a medical convention, I had a conversation with Kris Kuipers, a fellow passenger. He and I were commenting on the professionalism displayed by a flight attendant assigned to the flight. During the conversation, he asked if I was familiar with the Delta Air Lines "one-question survey" of client satisfaction. When I answered that I was not, Kris shared it with me.

The Delta representative is instructed to ask, "Would you hire the person with whom you've just spoken?"

It is a good model for facial surgeons to emulate. Ask patients if they would hire your employees. During medical training, doctors do not routinely learn how to operate a business or manage employees. Identifying, hiring, and training staff and associates to think as you think, embrace and exhibit the same work ethic, and treat patients and fellow staff members as you'd have them treated is one of those unwritten "secrets to success." Receiving compliments on one's staff is a critical indicator of how successful a doctor/surgeon is in managing the practice. The converse is also true.

If it is determined that a member of the staff is a detriment rather than an asset, a frank discussion of their patient encounter practices is called for. The exact reasons for the counseling session must be laid out (in the presence of a witness) and accurately recorded, by both the doctor and the witness, in the employee's personnel file.

Once the "industry-wide process" of corrective action has been exhausted, it is in everyone's best interest that the noncompliant employee be terminated, "for cause." One should consult the legal and governmental requirements to avoid unnecessary and unfounded counterclaims. The bottom line is this: do not tolerate a less than stellar staff. A facial surgeon can—and must—have an extraordinary support team.

Unequivocally, first impressions count. From the moment a prospective patient makes the initial contact with a facial surgeon (whether it be through a Web site, a phone call, or an encounter out in the community), in the prospective patient's mind, they begin to develop a profile of the surgeon, the staff, and the environment in which care is provided.

The geographic location of a facial surgeon's office, the external appearance of the building and grounds, interior furnishings, accessories, art, and music playing in the background create an impression (ambiance)—a positive impression or one of a negative nature. A good impression is easily built upon, whereas a negative first impression must be overcome. It is strongly recommended that the facial surgeon consult with a reputable architect/designer when planning the site of practice. For the surgeon already in practice, it might be helpful to consult with a designer about making changes to the existing décor/ambiance.

To see what patients see, from time to time doctors should visit their waiting room. They should also place a phone call to the reception desk from an outside phone periodically to see how the telephone is answered and listen to "on hold" music or recordings. Music played within the office or on a telephone can set a positive or negative stage of ambience.

When attempting to create a positive impression, one should avoid anything that could potentially be offensive to a customer/patient. Soft background music is recommended for facial surgery offices and clinics.

Public areas within a medical/surgical office are not appropriate places to display sports memorabilia and fan-based colors. There are private places (out of the sight of patients) in every office/clinic for such items.

Reading materials and video entertainment should be offered in good taste. It is perfectly appropriate to have a closed-circuit video production about the doctors and examples of work performed.

In waiting areas hardcover books are recommended over magazines, which become ragged and often have advertisements torn from the pages. Certificates, diplomas, promotional brochures, and pamphlets should be tastefully displayed.

If prospective patients are given the impression that the doctor/surgeon does not pay close attention to their office setting and staff, the natural assumption is that they do not pay close attention to other matters.

4 The Image of an Elite Facial Surgeon

The image a physician builds within the community and among colleagues is an asset, one to which a value cannot be tangibly applied. In the Author's Note at the front of this book, I referenced an admonition offered by Dr. Tinsley Harrison. About the calling that befalls a physician (including facial surgeons), Dr. Harrison offered the challenge to "provide a unique service for [one's] fellowman" and—at the same time—"build an enduring edifice of character" within oneself. The words *unique service* in Dr. Harrison's challenge are another way to say "distinguished" or "elite."

Clearly, the ultimate objective must be to build an edifice through "service." At the same time, ethical marketing practices can tastefully introduce the appearance–enhancement surgeon to the public and members of one's profession. To some of our colleagues it may sound strange, but professionals have one commodity to offer—what they know, and what they can do with what they know. And the more accessible that commodity/asset becomes to the public, the greater its value.

Accepting this contemporary truism to be valid, marketing facial surgeons and their practices has become big business—"mainstream" continuing medical education (CME). Virtually every CME conference contains segments of the program devoted to the subject.

It is not the intent of this chapter—or this book—to provide counseling on specific marketing techniques and campaigns, but rather to address marketing as part of practice development to be considered with forethought and entered into with prudence and good taste.

Social media plays a role in marketing exposure and will be addressed in the next chapter. First, however, I focus on something usually overlooked by marketing experts—the one-on-one, face-to-face encounter.

While establishing a public image (regardless of the credentialing pathway chosen by the physician), first impressions matter. With this fact at the forefront of their mind, aspiring facial surgeons must be aware of the image that comes to mind whenever and wherever they are seen, or when their name is spoken. Is the image one of

- Professionalism and respect?
- Community involvement?
- Being a good citizen?
- Sharing one's talents, knowledge, and resources to make the community a better place?
- Being a good husband, father, boss, and role model?

Or is it the antithesis of the above?

The right kind of visibility cannot be overstated, especially during the development years of one's practice, and in reminding colleagues and prospective patients that one is still actively practicing facial surgery.

When placed in a positive light, it is difficult to place a value on name recognition—and repetition. And there are several respectable ways to build name recognition and create the kind of positive image that appeals to the community, without having to pay exorbitant prices. It all begins with appearing approachable and having a heartfelt commitment to give as much back to the community as one takes from it. Here are a few ways to create a positive public image:

- Become active in civic clubs, faith-based groups, institutions, and charitable organizations.
- Volunteer to coach youth teams and participate in school activities.
- Become an active member of the area's chamber of commerce and Better Business Bureau.
- Volunteer to help out at local schools and school-related activities.
- Participate in athletic-oriented activities. Participate in golf, tennis, and handball tournaments, as well as runs, walks, biking events, and so forth that raise money for the underprivileged and underserved.
- Attend class reunions and homecomings. Let former classmates know about the nature of your practice and where it is located. And behave as a professional during such outings.
- Become involved in—and support—cultural institutions and activities within the community (museums, symphonies, opera, ballet, etc.).
- Be nice to everyone—hospital staff, servers, security guards, maintenance personnel, and checkout clerks. Everyone knows someone.

And then there is the social media aspect of creating and maintaining a positive professional image. The next chapter deals with that subject.

The takeaway message in this chapter is this: be visible—and recognizable—in very positive ways. At all times, avoid being where one ought not be, or with people with whom one ought not be associated. The old adage "One is known by the company one keeps" is one that should be at the forefront of the mind of a professional.

When approached or contacted by a prospective patient or a colleague who may wish to refer family members or patients, be attentive and considerate. Demonstrate appreciation that you are being considered, in a manner that does not appear solicitous. Never forget that you are a professional, offering your skills, knowledge, and empathy for fellow human beings as a service to humanity. In all areas of life, conduct yourself in a manner that builds upon the edifice of fellow physicians/surgeons who preceded you.

The preceding suggestions have proven to be effective in helping build a facial surgeon's public and professional image. Do not fail to connect this dot: building an elite practice begins with building a positive professional and public image. Once a positive image has been established, value it and protect it as the most prized possession you have—because it is!

5 The Role of Social Media

With David DeSchoolmeester

Social media is a must in any business today, and certainly for an elite facial surgery practice. It is beneficial for the surgeon who has an established practice *and more so* for the evolving practice.

In this chapter we recommend several social media avenues that have proven to be effective. First, however, we address *the message* a facial surgeon should be communicating with prospective patients, regardless of the methods.

An old marketers' saying deserves repeating here: "Features tell; benefits sell! "

Messaging involves more than discussing facial features. For example, consider the statement "During the procedure, your nose will be reduced in size." This message does not elicit an emotion. It requires more, such as addressing *the benefits* of having a procedure performed. Statements like these will go a long way toward convincing patients that this is something they really want to have: "Your nose will be more in harmony with other features, so that you will feel more confident." Or for patients above the age of 40, you might say, "People will notice how much younger you look with fewer sags and wrinkles." For any facial enhancement procedure, you might say, "When you exude more confidence in yourself, others will have more confidence in you." Describing *the benefits* of the procedure in your patient's life and what it will do for their morale, confidence, and overall emotional wellbeing is much stronger than just identifying the features you are qualified to enhance.

Next, we address the social media platforms that we believe provide the most benefit to your practice.

Then we will present testimonials from two young facial plastic surgeons who have recently entered private practice and whom I have asked to share some of their own experiences with social media. The first to weigh in will be Dr. W. Marshall Guy, a tech-savvy facial plastic surgeon who has a good grasp on social media networking. Dr. Guy is currently in private practice in the Woodlands community of the Houston, Texas, metropolitan area. After that we will turn to another doctor who trained with me at my institute. Dr. Parker A. Velargo practices in New Orleans, Louisiana, and limits his practice to facial plastic surgery. His partner practices comprehensive plastic surgery. Like Dr. Guy,

15

Dr. Velargo is extremely tech savvy. He has also agreed to share his experience in incorporating social media into a master practice–building initiative.

■ Testimonial from Dr. Guy

Facebook

The number one choice is no surprise here—Facebook. As a facial surgeon you should have *a business page* (in addition to whatever personal page you have) on Facebook, one specifically designed for your practice. Here you can list your hours of operation and locations and provide some basic information about your services, especially a link back to *your practice Web site.*

It is important to remember that Facebook is a *social* media site and you must learn to be "social" on it. That doesn't mean that you should spend hours on end engaging prospective patients here. You should make your page in keeping with that of a professional, but also fun and memorable.

There are two types of postings that should be included on your business Facebook page. An example of something fun is, maybe, every Tuesday your marketing person posts a picture of a famous person's eyes and your followers guess to whom the eyes belong. Then the following day, your marketing person posts the eyes, along with the entire face (same picture the eyes came from) side by side, as well as the correct answer.

Each famous person depicted should be someone who is generally thought of as a handsome man or a beautiful woman. Your pictures don't have to single out eyes though. Maybe the next week your marketing person picks a different person and instead of the eyes, the chin is shown, or maybe the mouth or nose. This may not sound like it pertains to your practice, but it does.

With each series of posts, you are sending subliminal messages to your followers. Showing perfect or near perfect features of famous people draws your followers' attention to their own features, for comparison.

Another kind of post might be a short (3- to 5-minute) video that teaches your audience something. The focus could be on answering frequently asked questions, at least in the beginning. That would transition into having your audience ask questions *for you* to answer. You must be very careful not to give specific advice in such a public setting. You can invite patients who wish specific advice to contact you directly. You should also have—and promote—a link that goes back to your site. Ask your followers to like your video and share it with their friends.

Video is a more effective way to have your audience bond with you, get to know you, and most of all, trust you. And it *must* be you, the physician, performing in the video. You are the one they want to hear from, and you want them to trust and bond with you. These videos *will not* take up too much of your time.

You should be able to record 3 months' worth of videos in less than 2 hours. You should post one per week on top of the famous person fun posts at one per week.

When you begin to build an audience on Facebook, you should consider using *Facebook Live*, at least once each month. This does not have to be in addition to your weekly video posting for that week. It can replace it. This allows real-time viewing of you during which your audience can ask questions by posting to your live feed during the session. You can answer them in real time. As with any performance, practice the session first.

You or a member of your marketing team needs to post something at least weekly to keep your audience entertained. This may be answers to commonly asked questions, discussing new technologies or treatments, or simply providing general tips to help keep your clients looking their best. The key is consistency so that people know to anticipate and look for your post.

Share your professional page with all of your friends. It is a quick way to get some likes. When your friends see your posts they can like them and also share them, which then leads to a blossoming (or ripple) effect and elicits more views. The other way to get likes and visualization of your post is to pay for it. This method is faster and easier, but it costs money.

You can also highly select the audience that you want *based on demographics*, although this does add to the cost of marketing. Once you have the likes, you can then begin marketing to people who have already liked your page. This focuses your dollars on those already interested in your services, which makes the return on investment higher.

YouTube

YouTube postings take advantage of videos you have already recorded and performed—the same ones you used for Facebook. Different social media sites have different audiences. That this is true allows you to reach different demographics by repurposing the same content to several locations.

Make sure you include a description of the video's content and include the link to your practice Web site *at the top* of the description. It needs to be at the top of the description because when people view your YouTube video, they only see a very small part of the description. Viewers must expand the description section to see everything written there. Including the link back to your Web site at the top of the description ensures each viewer will see it immediately.

Besides the fact that YouTube is the second or third largest Internet search engine, *it is also owned by Google*. This will help you in your Web site placement on the Google search engine. Google likes it when you use companies they own. For the same reason, if you decide to have an external blog (one not hosted on your Web site), make sure you use blogger.com. Blogger is also owned by

Google. Your blog should be hosted on your own Web site to give your audience the same look and feel as the rest of your site. Again, reuse your same video content here in your blog.

LinkedIn

LinkedIn is another very large social media site. It has similar methods to post your articles and video content, *and* it reaches yet another demographic, a more "professional" crowd, a demographic that is likely to react favorably to your messaging.

These three social media sites—Facebook, YouTube, and LinkedIn—will usually serve an elite facial practice. All have very good marketing tools that allow you to pinpoint your target audience. Of course there may be some overlap of audiences served by these three sites, but facial surgeons using them will have no problem reaching the bulk of individuals who either want or need their services.

iTunes

One more location should be considered. iTunes has a huge audience; and people who listen to or watch podcasts don't necessarily spend a lot of time on the top social media sites already listed. Having a podcast "show" brings with it even more credibility and authority. The availability of podcast sessions can also become a standard feature on your Web site.

Once again, the same videos you created for other social media outlets can be used in your podcast show.

So a social presence on the Internet will not take as much time as you might think. The content is created once and used in each of the locations—Facebook, YouTube, LinkedIn, and iTunes. Each time it reaches a different section of the population that would respond to your message.

Social marketing is really the lifeblood of a new practice. For those who are more established, it helps to keep patients and recruit more. But for those who are just opening their facial plastic surgery practice, it is an absolute must.

The questions arise how, what, and where to engage in social marketing. Unfortunately, there is no magic bullet that works for everyone, and in different markets different media will be more effective.

Twitter

Twitter is another medium for social marketing. Twitter is a microblogging site that allows you to send out messages to your followers. To keep your audience engaged, you really need to be putting out tweets more frequently than your

Facebook posts, daily if possible. Twitter is a nice medium for getting out information quickly to your followers. Unlike Facebook, where your posts may or may not be seen by your audience, your tweets will go out to all of your followers. Whether they read them or not is up to them, but they can at least see that you sent them out.

Instagram

The last social medium I wanted to comment on is Instagram. Being that our field is visual, this can be a great source of marketing. It does carry with it the most liability to make sure you are HIPAA compliant, but it is a great way for your followers to post about their experience with you. When *the patient is posting* it is (supposedly) not in violation of HIPAA, but double-check with your legal team. Because your patients can see you in your photos, it is a great way to keep people engaged.

Blogs

Finally, on your own Web site, you can include a *blog*. This is a great way to keep all of your Facebook posts, tweets, and photos in one place. There are also services that can automatically populate each of your social media posts for you (so you can have one post or announcement that goes to all of them and is also archived on your blog).

Summary

The key with all of social media marketing is *content*. Creating original content is ideal because it separates you from the pack. Anyone can pay a marketing company to post canned items. This will not improve your rankings on search engines, but it is one way of delegating the social media aspect. But if you really want to engage your audience, *write the posts yourself*. The great thing is you can write a lot of posts ahead of time and schedule them.

Whether you are a fan of social media or not, it is an integral part of a successful practice. Learning the basics, creating original content, and keeping your audience engaged truly can make or break your practice.

■ Testimonial from Dr. Velargo

Social media has become a progressively popular platform to promote one's practice in facial plastic surgery and plastic surgery. It is arguably the most powerful way to reach thousands of individuals who otherwise would never have heard of one's practice for free.

While the early times of social media favored usage by younger patients, the demographics of social media usage have changed. According to Pew,[1] young adults (ages 18 to 29) are the most likely to use social media (90%), but usage among those 65 and older has more than tripled since 2010 (35%). Usage in those age 30 to 49 (77%) and 50 to 64 (51%) has also increased over time. These demographic changes play positively to the facial plastic surgeon and plastic surgeon alike. With the increase in usage by older individuals, the surgeon may now sensibly promote procedures that target patients with aging face concerns. Additionally, older patients can usually afford appearance-enhancing surgery. Even so, younger patients still comprise the majority of social media users. The American Academy of Facial Plastic and Reconstructive Surgery noted a whopping 64% increase in cosmetic surgery or injectable treatments in patients under age 30 in 2015.[2]

My own practice currently participates on seven social media platforms: Facebook, Twitter, Google Plus, Instagram, Pinterest, LinkedIn, and RealSelf. We are currently setting up an account on the newest social media platform, Snapchat. Each of these platforms has unique characteristics, so they cannot be treated equally. An often unspoken advantage of all social media platforms is that one can "keep an eye" on the competition. Seeing new products or procedures that local plastic surgery practices are offering, as well as pricing and specials, is particularly useful in identifying where one stands in the community.

Facebook

Facebook is perhaps the most well known and utilized of the social media platforms. While many facial surgery practices may obtain tunnel vision and only focus on the number of likes that the practice's page gains, having a Facebook presence is much more than this. It creates brand awareness and allows followers to see the personality of one's practice in their daily news feeds. Facebook has also created ways for one's practice to create relatively inexpensive paid ads, targeted at a very particular audience (e.g., women ages of 30–50 who like Prada and The Real Housewives and live within a 10-mile radius of New Orleans, Louisiana). The ads target all individuals who meet the criteria regardless of whether they like your page or not. The price for such ads is determined by how many "impressions" or views your ad receives. Facebook allows you to reach many more users than those who like your business, which is also a great benefit. For example, if one of your followers likes a post on your news feed, then all of their "friends" will see the like, which allows for an exponential exposure, or "reach," as Facebook calls it. Facebook also allows users to rate your practice and write a review on your page.

As with all social media, one must exercise caution with Facebook in regard to HIPAA compliance because real names are used on this platform. While your patients may be willing to engage with the content of your page and divulge their treatments, the practice must refrain from revealing what treatments the patients have had or are planning to have. Facebook has generated a moderate amount of new referrals to my practice; moreover, many patients have claimed offers that are placed solely on our Facebook page. I find Facebook an extremely useful tool.

Twitter

Twitter is a fast "what's happening" application, which limits "tweets" (posts) to 140 characters. This means you have to get creative to stay under this limit and also post often to stay relevant. Twitter is a great platform to share deals and discounts or announce sales and new products. People use the hashtag symbol (#) before a relevant keyword or phrase in their tweet to categorize those tweets and help them show up more easily in a Twitter search. Hashtags are also popular tools in Facebook, Instagram, Pinterest, and Google Plus. Clicking or tapping on a hashtagged word in any message shows you other tweets that include that hashtag (all users, not just ones that follow you or that you follow). For example, searching for #plasticsurgery or #botox will generate thousands of tweets that mention these categorized words. This allows you to see what is trending, which may influence your current practice specials or promotions.

Google Plus (Google+)

Google+ has the distinct advantage of increasing your Google visibility and helping customers find your business faster. The +1 button also increases the chance of this visibility, as the more +1's a link has, the more attention it gets in search results. Hashtags are also useful on Google+, and one can also post photographs on Google+. Your practice can also have live video chat sessions with followers through "Hangouts." Many times, my Google+ posts will have some redundancy with my Facebook posts, but I find it important to post on Google+ simply to achieve higher organic placement on Google searches.

Instagram

Instagram is a mobile photo and video sharing application. It is designed to be utilized from a mobile device, and unlike Facebook, Twitter, or Google+, each post must include a photo or video (on the others these are optional). This is a great platform to demonstrate nonsurgical or even surgical procedures, as well as before and after photographs, as long as appropriate patient consent is obtained. Hashtags are perhaps the most useful on this platform, since users can list up to 30 hashtags per post. Users often follow your account after seeing your posts under trending hashtags. This obviously builds your brand awareness and visibility over time.

Pinterest

Pinterest is a great social media platform to showcase photographs. Whether you are posting photographs of products, infographics, or before and after photographs, patients love to see images. Users and businesses have a main "board" where photos are categorized. Users search for various things, such as "plastic surgery" or "facelift," which takes them to every "pin" that every user/business has posted containing those words. Users may then "re-pin" your photographs on their board as a reference for future treatments or general interest. It is in your best interest to be detailed in your photo description with back links to your Web site to drive traffic to your site. Remember to obtain special consent prior to posting patient photographs.

LinkedIn

LinkedIn is limited in terms of patient recruitment and is mostly used for recruiting new staff or, more often, having other professionals contact your company regarding services that they offer. Doctors often post their resumes, publications, and skill sets on this site. It is of limited use unless you are looking for new employees or looking to connect with another professional who can offer you a service your company needs.

RealSelf

RealSelf is a plastic surgery–specific social media platform. It is the most useful social media platform in my practice, given that it generates the most new patient consults and conversions by far. Each physician has a RealSelf profile, which allows one to answer questions posed by actual patients across the world. Only physicians certified in a core aesthetic specialty may participate in this forum (plastic surgery, facial plastic surgery, otolaryngology, dermatology, and oculoplastic surgery/ophthalmology). Physicians may elect to purchase an advanced profile, which allows them to post practice specials and also allows the publication of the physician's Web site. Patients write reviews of physicians on this site and are allowed to interact with other patients as a plastic surgery community—supporting, educating, and reassuring each other.

In addition to question answers, doctors post videos and photos in an effort to educate patients on various procedures and illustrate with before and after photographs that are representative of their work. The more questions physicians answer, the more media they post, the higher their patient rating, and the more active they are, the higher they are placed when patients search for doctors performing a certain procedure in the "find a doctor" search tool. Additionally, patients may directly e-mail doctors questions or request consultations electronically through the site. While the primary goal is patient education, physicians can easily establish themselves as experts and build patient trust even before the initial consultation.

Snapchat

The newest social media tool is Snapchat. While I currently do not participate in Snapchat, our practice soon will. This application allows users to tune into one's practice and watch the physician perform surgery or other procedures. The clips do not have to be a certain size or be censored for nudity, which is not a problem for facial procedures. Once followers watch the clip, it is deleted from their account and can never be seen again.

Users may take screenshots of the videos, but the practice knows who does this and can block those users from watching the practice content if inappropriate. Many followers are interested in knowing how a procedure is performed and getting to know the physician's style and personality prior to pursuing the treatment themselves, so this is a great tool for them. Users may ask questions, and the interaction is quite educational. Some prominent surgeons claim a very significant increase in business (and fame) as a result of this application. Again, great care must be exercised with patient consent and HIPAA compliance.

Summary

With the plethora of social media platforms in use, it is becoming increasingly difficult for surgeons to manage all of them, in addition to their day-to-day practice. With the exception of RealSelf, it is advisable to hire help in managing this aspect of the practice and keeping you relevant in social media. Our practice utilizes the same marketing company that maintains our Web site for this purpose.

Snapchat will require even more help, given that videos will need to be filmed, edited, and uploaded. Remember, however, that one's skillful investment into these social media platforms will result in a higher patient consultation rate, recognition as an expert in your field among the patient community, greater brand awareness, and greater visibility and geographic reach. Social media is an absolutely essential part of any facial plastic surgery practice.

■ Conclusion

The input of a social media/practice–building authority and two facial surgeons who have actually converted *advice* into *results* should provide valuable guidance for any surgeon committed to establishing an elite facial surgery practice.

The takeaway message in this chapter is this: *be visible—and recognizable—in very positive ways.* At all times, conduct yourself as a professional, as though prospective patients are watching—because they are, especially when it comes to social media.

■ References

1   http://www.pewinternet.org/2015/10/08/social-networking-usage-2005-2015/
2   http://www.aafprs.org/media/stats_polls/m_stats.html

6 The Ever-Growing Attraction to Facial Surgery

To understand the profession with which you are (or are about to be) identified, you must understand the mind-set of the client/patient population you aspire to serve. It is in that vein that the following is offered.

Each year, the world over, millions of people undergo appearance-enhancing procedures. It is a way to "invest" in themselves—in improving their appeal index. A high percentage of these individuals are opting for procedures to reverse the visible signs of aging. Others undergo surgery designed to reconstruct a portion of the face that is not in harmony with its other features. Still others seek facial surgery to improve features deformed by an accident, tumor surgery, or a congenital defect.

A national survey (*Psychology Today*) indicates that 40% of Americans are dissatisfied with the shape of their noses and 25% are dissatisfied with their "chins" (really necks). Furthermore, 35% of all facial surgery is performed on men, and that percentage is increasing.

These are important facts that a facial surgeon can share with potential patients who may be teetering on whether surgery is right for them.

Enhancing one's appearance can open doors to interpersonal relationships that might have otherwise remained closed, including doors of opportunity within the workplace. In Chapter 10, I address how people who do all the things required to look their best tend to find—and enjoy—better health, longer workspans, and higher incomes.

America in the 21st century is a youth-oriented, competitive society with a strong emphasis on appearance. Irrespective of "political correctness," the business community seeks out attractive people to fill available positions. Those who have the responsibility of hiring new employees confirm that, when all other qualifications are equal, a pleasing appearance gives an applicant (or candidate for promotion) the advantage. A facial surgeon can help individuals from all walks of life improve upon their current station.

Although definitions of beauty have varied through the ages, the fact that favors are granted to individuals considered to be handsome or beautiful has never changed. But it goes farther back in history than the modern medical literature. Aristotle said, "Beauty is a better recommendation than any letter of introduction."

Is it any wonder that many patients who have appearance-enhancing procedures do so for economic reasons? This is true not only for the fashion model, television and movie personality, corporate executive, or professional person, but also for anyone whose work or lifestyle requires interaction with the public.

Not only do people in the upper socioeconomic bracket undergo appearance-enhancing procedures, but so do people living on a budget. Most people plan for their procedures as they plan for a vacation, a new piece of jewelry, or an automobile. Improving their appearance is viewed as an investment in themselves.

Today, many sources of financing are available for plastic surgery. I recommend caution in this practice. No person should embark on a procedure that they cannot realistically afford. The dental profession has a saying, "The happy denture is the one that is paid for." Facial surgeons can learn from other health care professionals. Especially when it comes to age-reversing surgery—and no matter who performs it—in a couple of years new aging can be detected in a person's face. I have heard it said by a patient who financed her facelift with a company that provides such services, "I don't have my first facelift paid off and already I'm beginning to see my face aging again." Rhinoplasties and facial implants are a different matter. The results of such procedures are long-lasting.

Teachers, from kindergarten to professional institutions, affirm the long-held belief that—in the classroom—appearance matters. Many have told me that the young people they teach relate better to them after they undergo facial rejuvenation procedures that narrow the generational gap.

On both sides of the equation, a pleasing appearance provides advantages. Renowned psychologist Dr. Perry Buffington affirmed that "good looks affect school grades." Furthermore, according to Dr. Buffington one's looks also "determine who will become our friends, and enhance the probability of prosperity."

Love, luck, confidence, fame, and fortune tend to favor the person who presents a more pleasing appearance. When one looks better, one's pride and ego are bolstered, and surprisingly enough, it has been shown that when one feels good about oneself, one performs better, in all areas of life. And the world notices.

Corporate America certainly understands the value Americans place upon personal appearance. Billions of dollars are spent each year by people from all walks of life on cosmetics, accessories, fashionable wardrobes, vitamins, health foods, and weight control products. Many of these same individuals also have plastic surgery and care for their skin.

Aesthetic skin care encompasses a variety of methods designed to improve the quality, texture, and health of the skin. Medical aestheticians can also serve as consultants on healthy cosmetics, age prevention, improved toning of the muscles of the face and neck, and some medical skin conditions.

The world in which we live is a highly competitive place. And those who thrive in such an environment understand not only how to survive, but also how to rise above the masses and above circumstances.

Facial surgeons have an opportunity to serve as life coaches. They are uniquely prepared to counsel patients without appearing solicitous in the process.

It is appropriate to inform patients that people (both male and female) who undergo an appearance-enhancement procedure also tend to

- Pay attention to their weight.
- Engage in physical activity that tones and strengthens muscles and improves cardiovascular health.
- Maintain hormones at levels consistent with those of youth.
- Visit a medical spa for relaxation and scientific skin care.
- Augment their diet with pharmaceutical-grade vitamins and supplements.
- Have their teeth whitened.
- Coordinate their clothes.
- Groom their hair.
- Engage in activities that enhance the mind and spirit, as well as the body.
- Associate with others who have adopted the same lifestyle habits.

Other facts should be shared with patients. Attractive people appear to be happy. And people who appear to be happy make others want to be in their presence. Regardless of age, attractive people are attracted to other attractive, and thus success-minded, people.

Facial surgeons deal with a high volume of people who are concerned about the undesirable signs and symptoms of aging. An in-depth understanding of this patient population will give one an edge over competitors.

Patients often ask if they are too young or too old to have surgery. Here is a way to answer the question. Every individual has two "ages": the chronological one and the biological one. One's "chronological age" is determined by how many years one has lived. One's "biological age" is a reflection of how old one's body actually is—and appears—in comparison to others who have lived the same number of years.

It is helpful to explain to patients that several factors determine whether one's biological and chronological age are in balance. To help determine a patient's biological age, I require preoperative laboratory testing and a note from the patient's personal physician. In patients over the age of 40 this includes an electrocardiogram.

The best advice is to rely on the patient's personal physician to determine if a patient is an acceptable candidate for elective aesthetic surgery.

Some patients with the chronological age of 60 years appear to be 70. Others with a chronological age of 60 appear to be 50, even those who have had no previous facial plastic surgery. Lifestyle and genome are contributing factors.

If it is determined that the patient is in good health—and cleared to go under "twilight anesthesia"—chronological age is irrelevant.

A patient's psychological health is equally important. Facial surgeons should become familiar with psychological disorders that exist in some patients seeking appearance-altering surgery. The ability to distinguish between neuroses and psychoses is crucial. An undetected psychosis could lead to months—or years—of misery for the surgeon.

Following surgery, most patients experience some degree of depression and anxiety about the healing process and outcome of the surgery. Knowing how to shepherd them through the process can further solidify the doctor-patient relationship.

Refer patients suspected of having body dysmorphic disorder to a psychiatrist before agreeing to perform any surgical procedure.

An experienced facial surgeon is usually able to determine if younger patients (children or teenagers) are psychologically mature enough to undergo a procedure that is appropriate for their biological and chronological age.

Chapter 9 is dedicated to the power of thought—mind over matter. The reason for this should be obvious. Regardless of a patient's biological or chronological age, a positive outlook on life cannot be underestimated. People who look for the good and positive in every situation tend to find whatever it is they seek. (They also tend to be easier patients to care for following surgery). In adulthood, those with a positive outlook usually appear—and act—younger than their chronological age. The reverse is also true.

A variety of factors are responsible for one's biological age. It is not necessary that facial surgeons become experts in comprehensive health care; however, they must remain familiar enough with the subject to recognize when it is advisable to refer a patient to colleagues who focus on wellness and well-being.

As referenced in Chapter 11, balanced nutrition (with the appropriate supplementation) is a major factor in maintaining one's weight and health and an ongoing attractive appearance.

Physical activity not only burns calories but also keeps circulation flowing and muscles strong. Weight-bearing exercise tends to keep bones strong and combats one of the "silent killers," osteoporosis. Consider this little-known fact: 90% of individuals over the age of 70 who fracture a hip (and suffer from osteoporosis) die within a year of the incident. Many patients who seek rejuvenation surgery are in this age group. This fact makes osteoporosis a major health risk, one that—with preventive measures—can be affected in a positive manner.

In Chapter 11, I also address the importance of maintaining balance with the body's hormonal system. I once consulted with a lady who had undergone a facelift and surgery to correct saggy/baggy eyelids just months previously. After spending a few minutes inquiring about health issues, I suspected that she suffered from a common condition in postmenopausal women—hypothyroidism.

A series of laboratory tests confirmed my suspicion. Photographs (**Fig. 6.1**) demonstrate her appearance before and after thyroid replacement therapy. No surgery was performed. Her pretreatment symptoms were fatigue, feeling cold, and forgetfulness, along with the signs of fluid retention, dry skin, and a puffy face and eyelids. All disappeared once thyroid levels were normalized. The result: her appearance was enhanced, as were her spirits and well-being.

This case emphasizes the importance of a facial surgeon fulfilling the role of a physician first—a surgeon second. Another surgical procedure was not what this lady needed. She needed the expert care of a fellow physician who was qualified to offer condition-specific therapy I could not offer.

This is the final teaching point of this chapter. No doctor can be all things to all people. We facial surgeons must recognize our limitations and reach out to colleagues who are better trained and more experienced in treating conditions with which we are not so familiar.

Referring a patient to a colleague is never viewed by the patient as a sign of weakness or incompetence. Rather, it is looked upon as the professional—and caring—thing to do. More often than not a professional referral enhances the image of the referring physician/surgeon.

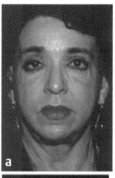
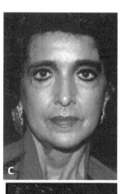
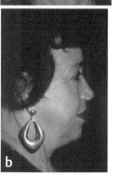
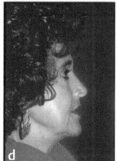

Fig. 6.1 **(a,b)** Prior to thyroid replacement. **(c,d)** After thyroid replacement.

7 The Enduring Doctor-Patient Relationship

Patients who seek the services of an aesthetic facial surgeon bring a unique set of circumstances to the consultation. Because they do not rely on the referral networks of third-party payers, patients are free to choose among a cadre of surgeons. Likewise, a surgeon who is not bound by a third-party contractual agreement is free to accept—or deny—treatment. This set of circumstances means that the decision to enter into a doctor-patient relationship is one of mutual consent, outside third-party interference. This is true whether the interceding party is a government agency or an insurance company.

During a presentation to a convention of doctors who specialize in aesthetic/cosmetic facial surgery, Chicago health care attorney Alex Thiersch said, "Vetting patients is the most important skill a facial surgeon will need." One of the primary objectives of this book is to assist aesthetic surgeons in acquiring that skill.

Depending upon how candidates arrive at the decision to consult with a particular surgeon, patients contemplating facial surgery may be divided into three general categories.

The first group comes through a word-of-mouth referral network. A friend, family member, or business associate has had an encounter with the surgeon and recommended them. These are the easy ones. The patient already knows a great deal about the surgeon and the surgeon's clinic, staff, and perioperative and postoperative care and—most importantly—has seen the outcome of the global system of care the surgeon and staff provide. Many already know the costs associated with the surgery in which they are interested.

The second group of patients is generally familiar with the surgeon and the clinic. They don't personally know anyone for whom the surgeon has cared, but they have heard or read "positive things" about the surgeon. This group requires more nurturing in the preoperative consultation session. To allay the anxiety associated with this concern, it is your task to explain (in layman's terms) why you recommend a particular course of treatment and the available alternatives to your recommendations, and to set the patient's mind at ease with facts. Explain the degree of pain and discomfort the patient can expect, and that medication will be available to handle pain and discomfort, if it should be an issue. And reassure the patient that the treatment plan you have recommended will not produce the tell-tale signs of overly aggressive surgery.

The third group is the smallest segment of consultations I see at this stage in my career. It will, however, comprise a larger segment for younger colleagues early in the development of their practices. This group of prospective patients often finds the facial surgeon through Internet or social media searches or a hospital or medical association "referral service" or responds to an advertisement, yellow pages listing, or public service educational program. Consults from this group generally provide lower returns on the investment of marketing resources and tend to be less reliable.

I once attended a presentation of an early pioneer in multimedia medical advertising. After 2 years and hundreds of thousands of dollars, the colleague's bottom line message was this: Aggressive advertising brought more consultations into the office, but when the marketing costs were factored in, the "return on investment" (ROI) was disappointing. More significantly, clients/patients who responded to his ads were likely to be swayed by someone else's marketing efforts for future care. The bottom line was that patient loyalty and long-term doctor-patient relationships were not created. High-volume practices mean that the doctor/surgeon spends less quality time with each patient—and thus the enduring doctor-patient relationship may never develop. It's a vicious cycle: The practice becomes dependent upon high volume. The ROI for each patient is reduced.

In my experience, every minute spent with the patient after a procedure has been performed equates to another procedure at some point during the relationship. It is not unusual for a patient to schedule a minor procedure to size up the surgeon. If exceptional care and attention is provided for minor things, the message is that the same can be expected for larger things.

Regardless of the method by which the patient consults with a surgeon, creating a relationship based upon mutual trust and respect is paramount.

In my experience, concerns over after-surgery appearances are one of the greatest hurdles to overcome. Many prospective facial surgery patients have seen high-profile individuals who underwent plastic surgery and barely resemble themselves.

It is the responsibility of surgeons to assure the new patient that the techniques they utilize are designed to create a "natural, unoperated" postoperative appearance and that they are going to do everything in their power to make the patient's experience as convenient and comfortable as possible, and to deliver on the promises.

This next admonition will be a challenge for the average young facial surgeon. Never—ever—allow money to drive your recommendations for a patient. Here, I call upon the sage advice of one of my afore-referenced mentors, Dr. Jack Anderson. He said, "A good deal is a good deal for all parties. If either party senses they have been taken advantage of, the deal will fall apart." So the secret to establishing a long-term doctor-patient relationship is to make every encounter a "good deal" for all parties.

Along the U.S. Gulf Coast, there is a term that originated within the Cajun communities of Louisiana: *lagniappe*. It means "a little something extra; a bonus, for which the customer was not required to pay." I label this phenomenon the lagniappe principle. Offer patients something—at no "extra charge"—that they were not anticipating. But make sure it is clear beforehand that it is included in the "deal."

During a consultation with a prospective patient, should the patient feel that the surgeon is attempting to pile on procedures or that the charges quoted are exorbitant, the doctor-patient relationship falls apart, before it began.

Early in the consultation, point out good features of the patient's face and explain that no treatment is required at this time in those areas. Doing so gives the impression that the surgeon is not out to sign the patient up for more than is currently indicated. I use the following words: "This is good right now. We don't need to do anything about it at this time. We'll get around to it in a few years." This statement plants the seed for a long and mutually fruitful doctor-patient relationship. Regardless of how the prospective patient was directed to the facial surgeon's office, the objective during the first encounter should be uniquivocal: to create a professional relationship nurtured by mutual trust.

Patients are much better informed today than when I began my own practice 4 decades ago. They have access to more information about available procedures. Many have reviewed blogs and Web sites that post critiques—good and bad—about the lot of professionals who provide appearance-altering procedures. Some candidates for surgery are quite specific in asking if the surgeon being consulted uses a particular technique, device, or implant. In some respects the Internet creates a more difficult consultation for contemporary facial surgeons. They must be prepared to logically explain why their treatment plan is different from one posted by a colleague on the Internet or recommended during a face-to-face encounter.

Emerging technology can also serve to assist the patient and the facial surgeon in assessing each other. Skype and FaceTime technology allows face-to-face conversations. If a patient requests this venue, I require the patient to send a series of photographs ahead of time. The reason is that camera lenses for computers and cellular telephones generally create distortions that make it difficult to assess the patient's facial features.

Video conferencing allows the surgeon to obtain a general impression of the patient's demeanor, interpret body language, and hear the patient express specific concerns and desires. With electronic encounters, however, the facial surgeon should emphasize to the patient—and note in the medical record—that recommendations offered during media encounters are preliminary in nature and that the final treatment plan will be made during an on-site, face-to-face encounter prior to treatment.

Along those same lines, the surgeon should explain to each patient that—once surgery is performed—the patient is encouraged to e-mail photographs during the healing process. Doing so is a modern-day convenience not available in years passed and—in many cases—prevents unnecessary travel for patients who live great distances from the operating surgeon's practice. Whether this kind of doctor-patient interchange is "telemedicine" and rises to the standard of "practicing medicine across state lines" is an open-ended question. I attest that patients appreciate the fact that they are given their surgeon's direct e-mail address, can express concerns at will, and can reasonably expect a response within hours. It is one more way to provide extraordinary care in a competitive marketplace.

In the vast majority of cases, patients heal well and return to presurgery activities within a matter of days. However, the doctor-patient relationship is tested when problems and complications arise. And the manner in which the surgeon addresses unforeseen—and unfortunate—circumstances can either abruptly end the relationship or solidify it beyond imagination.

Expressing genuine concern for the patient's condition and anxiety associated with it is the first order of business. If a problem exists, readily admit that it exists; then assure the patient that they will not be abandoned. Explain that after things settle down, corrective measures—if indicated—will be performed. Denying that a problem exists (if it does) causes the patient to lose confidence and seek remedy elsewhere and sets the stage for legal recourse.

Surgeons who initiate proactive measures in such situations will usually find patients to be appreciative, understanding, and willing to return for additional procedures, for decades to come. They will also often bring family, friends, and associates with them.

So the takeaway-message in creating and maintaining a positive doctor-patient relationship is to follow the Golden Rule. Do for the patient what you would want done if you or a member of your immediate family were the patient.

An ounce of genuine caring is worth more than a shipload of lame excuses.

8 Elite Care: Beyond the Face and Neck

The role of aesthetic surgery in the well-being of human beings has long been documented. To provide exceptional care, facial surgeons must be of the mind-set that the object of their attention is an extraordinary being. The human body and the mind that reigns over it meet that criterion. Thus, physicians devoted to enhancing face, body, mind, and soul must be aware of the symbiotic role each of them plays in the care of the whole.

A primary objective of aesthetic facial surgery is to reverse the unwanted *signs* of aging; however, the responsibility of the surgeon does not end there. Oftentimes a face that appears to be aging prematurely is a reflection of a failing state of well-being elsewhere in the body.

Some scientists believe that the human body is capable of living 120 years. If that is true, then why don't humans live that long? Perhaps it is because of the things the species does *not* do to ensure health and well-being, and the external appearances thereof.

From a self-preservation standpoint, it seems that humankind can be divided into three groups.

The McCollough Classification of Health Awareness

- Group 1 does not understand how the body or mind works and knows not what to do to take care of it.
- Group 2 knows what should be done, yet chooses not to do what they know they should do.
- Group 3 knows what to do and does what they can to take care of themselves and those they care for—and about.

The above classification system calls for another one—a system that describes health care providers.

- *Group 1:* doctors who focus on lengthening life spans.
- *Group 2:* doctors who focus on enhancing the quality of life.
- *Group 3:* doctors focused on enhancing *both* the quality and quantity (span) of life.

The elite aesthetic surgeon fits comfortably into group 3. It is your responsibility to see that your patients determine in which of the three groups they currently exist. If they find themselves in group 3 of the health awareness scale, this book will show you (the facial surgeon) how to encourage them to continue along the same pathway and become an even better person, physically, mentally, and spiritually. If the physician (or the patient) is not now in group 3, I hope to show you how to become a living example of how they can follow your lead. Such a mind-set begins with an appreciation of the creative evolution of the species we know as human beings.

■ A Marvelous Creation

For thousands of years humankind has tried to understand life, death, and everything in between. We have come to realize that the human body is a marvelous and beautiful "creation." We believe that it is "the temple of the soul." History records that this temple has been worshiped, abused, and mutilated, sometimes knowingly, sometimes unknowingly, oftentimes by others, sometimes by the individual encased within it.

As far back as the history of civilization can be traced, humankind has sought ways to understand who we are, and to become something different from what we are—to evolve. One of the quests of such understanding has been focused on finding ways to defy aging. Expeditions were launched to discover the mythical "fountain of youth." The search is still on. It could emerge from some genetic scientist's laboratory.

Perhaps we have made some progress. In the 21st century, the life span of humans who practice "wellness lifestyles" is on the rise. People who adhere to healthy lifestyles are living longer. Conditions that cause us to die are changing. Obesity is the cause of much of the self-induced illness in Western civilizations.

Unlike many of our ancestors who died because of infections, childbirth, and accidents, more and more of us are dying of chronic diseases, many of which are self-inflicted as a result of the "seven deadly sins": hubristic pride, greed, lust, malicious envy, gluttony, uncontrolled anger, and sloth. These harmful characteristics of human behavior run counter to the "seven virtues": prudence, justice, temperance (meaning restriction or restraint), courage (or fortitude), faith, hope, and charity (or love). When incorporated into one's behavior and habits, these virtues may actually reduce the harmful aspects of stressful living and promote health and well-being.

As a result of the "information renaissance," we humans are learning more about ourselves. We are beginning to understand what enhances our bodies and minds and what tears them down.

Scientists are beginning to realize what James Allen and Dr. Orison Marden knew a century ago—that today many of the conditions that cause people to age and die we bring upon ourselves. The things we do (as well as the things we *do not* do) to our bodies either help the body to ward off disease or invite disease and premature aging. In that respect *we are a creator of our own state of health (and appearance)*, especially when we begin to view aging as a preventable and treatable disease.

A problem in the quest for perpetual youth is that it is difficult to determine the practical "age" of the human body. The reason is that our bodies keep time by *two* "clocks." One is the *chronological* clock, which records the number of years a person has lived. The other is the *biological* clock; it measures how "old" (senescent) the body actually is. The rate at which one's biological clock ticks is dependent on one's genetic makeup and thought processes and on the lifestyle choices one makes. Although we can't alter the chronological clock, it is possible to slow down or speed up one's biological clock.

■ Researching "Miracle" Treatments

In Western civilizations, there is a growing interest in programs, services, and products designed to help keep us young. The icons of health and beauty that adorn the covers of magazines and picture screens raise the bar, often to unrealistic levels. Even so, the public is actively seeking advice and treatment from doctors and allied health professionals. And it is often taken advantage of.

Almost everywhere you turn there is a "quick fix," a "simple" and "noninvasive" way to keep you young and fit. Remember the time-honored advice that *if it sounds too good to be true, it usually is.*

Aesthetic surgeons are in a good position to warn patients that when they are considering whether to purchase the "miracle" treatment of the month, they need to do the research. It is important to make sure that the services and products one is considering are grounded in science and can stand the test of validity.

■ Stopping Aging: Facts and Myths

With the growing commercialization of the health and beauty industry, the public is being bombarded with misinformation. One of the purposes of this book is to demystify some of what patients and colleagues alike are being told, and sold, so that facial surgeons can counsel patients in such matters.

Some of the terms used to describe the "rejuvenating and invigorative health sciences" are confusing and perhaps misleading. I have pointed out to my colleagues that the term *antiaging medicine* is—within itself—a misnomer, that to "antiage" is impossible. To slow, repair, rejuvenate, and invigorate is possible.

First, it is important for facial surgeons to understand (and explain to patients) that there is a difference between aging and being "old." Age is, to a great extent, a state of mind. Feeling and acting old is a choice. So is feeling, acting, and looking youthful, at any age.

Senescence is the term used to describe the physical and mental manifestation of being old. The word *senility* comes from the same root word.

On the other side of life's equation, "youth" is largely a state of mind.

"Rejuvenation" is the physical and mental manifestation of preserving or recapturing the mind-set of being young, and at the same time, invigorating and enhancing the body a person has at the time. Feeling and looking younger can be achieved regardless of how many years you may have lived. And it is to this side of life's equation that doctors, allied health professionals, and clients of rejuvenating physicians and surgeons must redirect part of the focus.

The objective in helping people look, feel, and perform better *is not to stop aging*. As simplistic as it may seem, *to stop aging is to die.* A more realistic objective is to accept the fact that—from the moment of birth—every human body continues to age (chronologically). The focus has to be redirected toward living as many years as possible, but to do so with a longer and vitality-filled "health span" and to look as youthful as one feels.

■ Experiencing Re-creation

In the quest to keep you or your patients from losing the battle of *premature* aging and help you focus thoughts and actions toward disease prevention and life enhancement, let us, first, agree on a few basic facts:

- Each body comprises many moving parts that are interdependent. It is, in fact, a biological "machine," which to perform at its maximum potential, must be cared for, maintained, and polished with pride and respect.
- Like the bodies of other living creatures, human bodies have a unique ability to adapt to circumstances and surroundings, whether the stimulus is of external or internal origin. And because of this, the body is in a constant state of change. It is the most evolved creation on Earth; yet it is being *re-created* cell by cell, day by day, and year by year. Many of us learned about this process in high school biology. It is called mitosis—a cell divides to produce a replica of itself.

- Since the delicate process of re-creation is ongoing, the care of one's body and mind becomes one's own responsibility as a body owner. That being the case, it is up to each individual, as the keeper of their "temple," to do everything within their power to protect it, maintain it, and whenever appropriate, adorn and enhance it.
- It is the responsibility of body owners to choose doctors and allied health professionals who can help them take care *of them*. It is also a doctor's responsibility to refer patients to a colleague who focuses on wellness to assist in the rejuvenation treatment plan, someone who will cheer them on as they defy the aging process and who will lend a helping hand when needed.

■ The Depths of Beauty and Handsomeness

For centuries, humankind has lived by the paradigm "Beauty is only skin deep." In the 21st century, however, that age-old adage is being challenged. The challenge is taking place because the physical and psychological relationship between appearance and health is emerging as a medical specialty unto itself. At the turn of the century, I named it "Rejuvenology," and I define it as "the scientific pursuit of the health, vitality, and youthful appearance that generally exist during the prime of human life."

Medical Rejuvenology uses nonsurgical means to enhance the human body. *Surgical Rejuvenology* (plastic surgery) changes the size, shape, and contours of body parts in ways that diet and exercise cannot. Aesthetic surgeons are, by definition, rejuvenologists. Best results are often obtained when both branches of the specialty are employed.

Rejuvenologists help patients get in touch with who they really are, inside and out. Once individuals have a clear understanding of who they are, they can see how they measure up to the person they wish to be. Then they can develop a personalized lifestyle prescription designed to help them become a better version of themselves. They will learn the true meaning of "optimal health" as it applies to them and their circumstances.

■ "Health" Defined

The World Health Organization defines "health" as "a dynamic state of complete physical, mental, spiritual, and social well-being and not merely the absence of disease or infirmity."

Rejuvenologists can help patients achieve a more advanced level of well-being, even if they have an existing health problem. And while perfection may be the lofty aspiration that facial surgeons will attempt to achieve, improvement is a more realistic goal.

In the sections that follow, you will become more familiar with how the two new branches of surgical and nonsurgical Rejuvenology are inseparable. You will see how both can help you maximize your own potential and help patients enjoy the longer, more productive life that you will help them create. You will help them see how what is happening *within their body* can now be examined and modified in ways previously thought impossible. You will provide guidance in how to become their own advocate in the arena of health and appearance enhancement. In short, you are about to become a partner in taking care *of your patient's* face, mind, body, and spirit.

As an elite facial surgeon, your task extends beyond taking care of a patient's face. It is to help those you care for do an even better job of caring for themselves.

■ Inside and Out

It is true that the way people look on the outside says a lot about them. However, advanced diagnostic testing methods have proven that it is not always possible to look at a person and tell if everything is optimal inside. So health care professionals must look to additional technology, which allows us to "look" *within and beneath the skin and into body cavities, organs, and blood vessels.* In reality, medical professionals have already achieved a major portion of that goal.

Many of my aesthetic surgery patients feel better because deficiencies in their diet and supplement programs and hormone levels were identified and corrected.

It is "good medicine" to empower patients with the knowledge, protocols, and procedures they need to become their own advocates in a personal journey toward achieving optimal health and appearance enhancement.

Advanced testing helps doctors determine if the body's intricate chemical and nutritional systems are balanced, not only within the blood fluids, but also within the cells, at a molecular level.

The point to remember is to recommend that a patient undergo the appropriate testing, and then follow through with whatever abnormality might be discovered. Emphasize that the vast majority of people who are tested leave with the peace of mind that nothing of any great importance was found. Most only need to adjust their eating and supplement habits and engage in more physical activity. Others recognize the need to learn how to manage the stresses of their everyday lives.

■ Keeping Connected

For individuals to be healthy, they must think healthy. In order for individuals to be attractive, they must feel attractive. Then, thoughts must be put into action and become good habits—age-defying, health-enhancing, life-enhancing habits.

9   The More Abundant Life

No one expresses the mind-body connection better than early 20th century physician and noticer Dr. Orison S. Marden. In *Peace, Power, and Plenty* he reveals the secret to a life of abundance—of youthful well-being.[1]

I offer Dr. Marden's ideology here for two reasons: for the well-being of the face-enhancing surgeon, and so that members of the profession can imbue these truisms into the minds of their patients. Doing so will help facial surgeons maintain their own heath, prolong career spans, obtain extraordinary outcomes, and provide a level of care not routinely offered throughout the appearance-enhancing industry. Readers who have not experienced the signs and conditions of aging should also heed the admonitions expressed in this chapter. The day will come when they will apply to you. In the meantime, you can help your patients slow the aging process. That you do will set you—and your practice—apart from other surgeons.

I summarize Marden's remarks. My own thoughts are parenthesized. For emphasis, some words and sentences are italicized.

Few people realize how largely their health (and appearance) depends upon the saneness of their thinking. You cannot hold ill thoughts, disease thoughts (old-age thoughts), in the mind without having them "out-pictured" in the body. *The thought will appear in the body somewhere.*

The health stream, if polluted at all, is polluted at the fountainhead—in the thought, in the ideal. We can never reach perfection by dwelling upon imperfection, harmony by dwelling upon discord (or youth by dwelling on aging).

We should keep a high ideal of health (youth) and harmony constantly before the mind. *Never affirm or repeat about your health (or appearance) what you do not wish to be true.*

The mind is the health and appearance sculptor, and we cannot surpass the mental pattern (upon which our minds focus). If there is a weakness or a flaw in the thinking model, there will be corresponding deficiencies in the health-statue.

We (facial surgeons) take infinite pains and spend many years in preparing ourselves for our lifework. We know that a successful career must be based upon scientific principles of training, of system and order, that every step of a successful career must be taken only after great thought and consideration. We know that it means years of hard work to establish ourselves in life in a profession or business; but our health, upon which everything else hangs—upon which it depends absolutely—we take very little trouble to establish.

When we remember that the integrity and efficiency of all the mental faculties depend upon health and that robust health multiplies 10-fold the power of our initiative, increases our creative ability, generates enthusiasm and spontaneity, and strengthens the quality of judgment, the power of discrimination, the force of decision, and the power of execution, we should be very diligent to establish it.

We (facial surgeons) should lay a foundation for our health just as we establish anything of importance—by studying and adopting the sanest and the most scientific methods. We should think health, talk health, hold the health ideal, just as a law student should think law, talk law, read law, live in a law atmosphere. Thinking is building; our thinking will be reflected in our bodies (and in the bodies of our patients).

Thoughts are things, and they leave their characteristic marks on the mind. Every true, beautiful, and helpful thought is a suggestion that, if held in the mind, tends to reproduce itself there—clarifies the ideals and uplifts the life. While these inspiring and helpful suggestions fill the mind, their opposites cannot put in their deadly work, because the two cannot live together. They are mutually antagonistic, natural enemies. One excludes the other.

The human body is made exclusively of cells. We are nothing but a mass of cells of 12 different varieties, such as brain cells, bone cells, and muscle cells. The maximum of health and power depends upon the absolute integrity of every cell. Sickness and disease simply mean that some of the cells in the body are impaired.

Many people seem to think that thought only affects the brain; but the fact is *we think all over.*

The body is a sort of extended brain. Every thought that enters the brain cells is quickly communicated to every cell in the entire body, thus accounting for the tremendous instantaneous influence of a shock caused by fatal news or some terrible catastrophe on every part of the body, instantly affecting all the secretions and functions. When the diseased thought goes, the body at once rebounds and becomes normal.

A short time ago I read a story about a young officer in India who consulted a great physician because he felt fagged from the excessive heat and long hours of service. The physician examined him and said he would write to him the next day. The letter the patient received informed him that his left lung was entirely gone and his heart was seriously affected, and it advised him to adjust his business affairs at once. "Of course, you may live for weeks," it said, "but you had best not leave important matters undecided."

Naturally the young officer was dismayed by this death warrant. He grew rapidly worse, and in 24 hours respiration was difficult and he had an acute pain in the region of the heart. He took to his bed with the conviction that he would never rise from it. During the night he grew rapidly worse and his servant sent for the doctor.

"What on earth have you been doing to yourself?" demanded the physician. "There was no indication of this sort when I saw you yesterday."

"It is my heart, I suppose," weakly answered the patient in a whisper.

"Your heart!" repeated the doctor. "Your heart was all right yesterday."

"My lungs, then," said the patient.

"What is the matter with you, man? You don't seem to have been drinking."

"Your letter, your letter!" gasped the patient. "You said I had only a few weeks to live."

"Are you crazy?" said the doctor. "I wrote you to take a week's vacation in the hills and you would be all right."

The patient, with the pallor of death in his face, could scarcely raise his head from the pillows, but he drew from under the bedclothes the doctor's letter.

"Heavens, man!" cried the physician. "This was meant for another patient! My assistant misplaced the letters."

The young officer sat up in bed immediately, and was entirely well in a few hours.

We are all at some time in our lives victims of the imagination. We are just beginning to appreciate the marvelous power of suggestion to uplift or depress the mind (and, thus, body).

When we are thoroughly entrenched in the conviction of our unity with the All-good, when we realize that we do not take on health from outside by acquiring it, but that we are health, then we shall really begin to live.

Multitudes of people undoubtedly shorten their lives by many years because of their deep-seated conviction that they will not live beyond a certain age—the age, perhaps, at which their parents died. How often we hear this said: "I do not expect to live to be very old; my father and mother died young."

If you have convinced yourself, or if the idea has been ingrained into the very structure of your being by your training or the multitudes of examples about you, that you will begin to show the marks of age at about 50, that at 60 you will lose the power of your faculties and your interest in life, that you will become practically useless and have to retire from your business (practice), and that thereafter you will continue to decline until you are cut off entirely, there is no power in the world that can keep the *old-age processes and signs* from developing in you.

Thought leads. If it is an old-age thought, old age must follow. If it is a youthful thought, a perennial young-life thought, a thought of usefulness and helpfulness, the body must correspond. *Old age begins in the mind.* The expression of age in the body is the harvest of old-age ideas that have been planted in the mind. We see others about our age beginning to decline and show marks of decrepitude, and we imagine it is about time for us to show the same signs. Ultimately we do show them, because we think they are inevitable. But *they are only inevitable because of our old-age mental attitude and beliefs.*

If we actually refuse to grow old, if we insist on holding the youthful ideal and the young, hopeful, buoyant thought, the old-age earmarks will not show themselves.

The elixir of youth lies in the mind or nowhere. You cannot be young by trying to appear so, by dressing youthfully. You must first get rid of the last vestige of thought that you are aging. As long as that is in the mind, cosmetics and youthful dress will amount to very little in changing your appearance. (For the rejuvenation surgery you perform on your patients to achieve its intended goals) the conviction (of being "old") must first be changed; the thought that has produced the aging condition must be reversed.

If we can only establish the perpetual-youth mental attitude, so that we feel young, we have won half the battle against old age. Be sure of this, that *whatever you feel regarding your age will be expressed in your body.* (And share these thoughts with your patients at every opportunity. Lead by example.)

It is a great aid to the perpetuation of youth to learn to *live young*, however long we may have lived, because the body expresses the habitual feeling, the habitual thought. Nothing in the world will make us look young as long as we are convinced that we are aging.

Nothing else more effectually retards age than keeping in mind the bright, cheerful, optimistic, hopeful, buoyant picture of youth in all its splendor and magnificence, the picture of the glories that belong to youth—youthful dreams, ideals, and hopes, and all the qualities that belong to young life.

One great trouble with us (humans) is that our *imaginations age prematurely.* The hard, exacting conditions of our modern, strenuous life tend to harden and dry up the brain and nerve cells and thus seriously injure the power of the imagination, which should be kept fresh, buoyant, elastic.

People who take life too seriously, who seem to think everything depends upon their own individual efforts, whose lives are one continuous grind in living-getting, have a hard expression; their thought out-pictures itself in their faces. These people dry up early in life, become wrinkled; their tissues become as hard as their thought.

The arbitrary, domineering, overbearing mind also tends to age the body prematurely, because the thinking is hard, strained, abnormal.

People who live on the sunny and beautiful side of life, who cultivate serenity, do not age nearly so rapidly as do those who live on the shady, the dark, side.

Another reason why so many people age prematurely is because they cease to grow. It is a lamentable fact that multitudes of humans seem incapable of receiving or accepting new ideas after they have reached middle age. Many of them, after they have reached the age of 40 or 50, come to a standstill in their mental reaching out.

Nothing else is easier than for people to age. All they have to do is to think they are growing old; to expect it, fear it, and prepare for it; to compare themselves with others of the same age who are prematurely old and to assume that they are like them.

The very belief that old age is settling upon us and that our life forces are gradually ebbing away has a blighting, shriveling influence upon the *mental* faculties and functions; the whole character deteriorates under this old-age belief.

The result is that we do not use or develop the age-resisting forces within us. The refreshening, renewing, resisting powers of the body are so reduced and impaired by the conviction that we are getting on in years and cannot stand what we once could, that we become an easy prey to disease and all sorts of physical infirmities.

The mental attitude has everything to do with the hastening or the retarding of the old-age condition.

Dr. Metchnikoff of the Pasteur Institute in Paris says that humans should live at least 120 years. There is no doubt that, as a race, we shorten our lives very materially through our false thinking, our bad living, and our old-age convictions.

It is an insult to our Creator that our brains should begin to ossify, that our mental powers should begin to decline when we have only reached the half-century milestone.

As long as you hold the conviction that you are 60, you will look it. Your thought will out-picture itself in your face, in your whole appearance. If you hold the old-age idea, the old-age conviction, your expression must correspond. The body is the bulletin board of the mind.

On the other hand, if you think of yourself as perpetually young, vigorous, robust, and buoyant, because every cell in the body is constantly being renewed, decrepitude will not get hold of you (and you will enjoy a long and gratifying career).

If you would retain your youth, you must avoid the enemies of youth. Nothing helps more in the perpetuation of youth than much association with the young.

A man quite advanced in years was asked not long ago how he retained such a youthful appearance in spite of his age. He said that he had been the principal of a high school for over 30 years, that he loved to enter into the life and sports of the young people and to be one of them in their ambitions and interests. This, he said, had kept his mind centered on youth, progress, and abounding life, and the old-age thought had had no room for entrance.

There is not even a suggestion of age in this man's conversation or ideas, and there is a life, a buoyancy, about him that is wonderfully refreshing.

Hold stoutly to the conviction that it is natural and right for you to remain young. Constantly repeat to yourself that it is wrong, wicked, for you to grow old in appearance. Constantly affirm, "I am always well, always young; I cannot grow old except by producing the old-age conditions through my thought. The Creator intended me for continual growth, perpetual advancement and betterment, and I am not going to allow myself to be cheated out of my birthright of perennial youth."

The great thing is to make the mind create the *youth pattern* instead of the *old-age pattern.* As the sculptor (or facial surgeon) follows the model that he holds in the mind, so the life processes reproduce in the body the pattern that is in our thought, our conviction. We must get rid of the idea embedded in our very nature that the longer we live, the more experiences we have, the more work we do, the more inevitably we wear out and become old, decrepit, and useless. We must learn that living, acting, experiencing, should not exhaust life but *create more life.*

Nature has bestowed upon us perpetual youth, the power of perpetual renewal. The body is constantly being made new through cell renewal, the cells of those parts of it that are most active being renewed oftenest. It must follow that the age-producing process is largely artificial and unnatural.

Physiologists tell us that the tissue cells of some muscles are renewed every few days, others every few weeks or months. The cells of the bone tissues are slower of renewal, but some authorities estimate that 80 or 90% of all the cells in the body of a person of ordinary activity are entirely renewed in from 6 to 24 months.

If the ideal of continual youth, of a body in a state of perpetual rejuvenation, dominates the mind, it neutralizes the aging processes. All of the body follows the dominating thought, motive, and feeling and takes on its expression. For example, a man (or woman) who is constantly worrying, fretting, a victim of fear, cannot possibly help out-picturing this condition in his (or her) body. Nothing in the world can counteract this hardening, aging, ossifying process but a complete reversal of the thought, so that the opposite ideas dominate. The effect of the mind on the body is always absolutely scientific. It follows an inexorable law: *as long as the mind faces the sun of life it will cast no shadow before it.*

Hold ever before you, like a beacon light, the youth ideal—strength, buoyancy, hopefulness, expectancy. Hold persistently to the thought that your body is the last 2 years' product, that there may not be in it a single cell more than a year and a half old, that it is constantly young because it is perpetually being renewed and that, therefore, it ought to look fresh and youthful. (As an appearance-enhancing surgeon, if you can imbue these thoughts into the minds of your patients, imagine how much better this added element of care will make your surgery appear.)

If you would keep young, you must learn the secret of self-rejuvenation, self-refreshment, self-renewal, in your thought, in your work. Hard thoughts, too serious thoughts, mental confusion, excitement, worry, anxiety, jealousy, and the indulgence of explosive passions all tend to shorten life.

Some people are so constituted that they perpetually renew themselves. They do not seem to get tired or weary of their tasks, because their minds are constantly refreshing themselves. They are self-renewers. To keep from aging, we must keep the picture of youth in all its beauty and glory impressed upon the mind. It is impossible to appear youthful, to be young, unless *we feel* young.

Without realizing it, most people are using the old-age thought as a chisel to cut a little deeper the wrinkles. Their old-age thought is stamping itself upon the new cells only a few months old, so that they very soon look to be 40, 50, 60, or 70 years old.

Never allow yourself to think of yourself as growing old. Constantly affirm, if you feel yourself aging, "I am young because I am perpetually being renewed; my life comes new every moment from the Infinite Source of life. I am new every morning and fresh every evening because I live, move, and have my being in Him who is the Source of all life." Affirm this not only mentally, but also verbally when you can. Make this picture of perpetual renewal, constant refreshment, re-creation, so vivid that you will feel the thrill of youthful renewal through your entire system. Under no circumstances allow the old-age thought and suggestion to remain in the mind. *Remember that it is what you feel, what you are convinced of, that will be out-pictured in your body. If you think you are aging, if you walk, talk, dress, and act like an old person, these conditions will be out-pictured in your expression, face, manner, and body generally. Youthful thought should be a life habit.*

Picture the cells of the body being constantly made over. Hold this *perpetual-renewal picture* in your mind, and the old-age thought, the old-age conviction, will become inoperative.

The new youth-thought habit will drive out the old-age-thought habit. *If you can only feel your whole body being perpetually made over and constantly renewed, you will keep the body young, fresh.* It is senility *of the soul* that makes people old.

The living of life should be a perpetual joy. Youth and joy are synonymous. If we do not enjoy life, if we do not feel that it is a delight to be alive, if we do not look upon our work as a *grand privilege*, we shall age prematurely.

Live in the ideal, and the aging processes cannot get hold of you. It is the ideal that keeps one young. Every time you think of yourself, make a vivid mental picture of your ideal self as the very picture of youth, of health and vigor. Feel the spirit of youth and hope surging through your body. Form the most perfect picture of physical manhood or womanhood that is possible to the human mind.

The elixir of youth that alchemists sought so long in chemicals we find lies in ourselves. The secret is in our own mentality. *Perpetual rejuvenation is possible only by right thinking. We look as old as we think and feel because it is thought and feeling that change our appearance.*

If we are convinced that the life processes can perpetuate youth instead of age, they will obey the command.

The body is simply a reflection of the mind; it cannot be anything else. It would be impossible for a person to hold only beautiful, loving thoughts in the mind and not have the body correspond and come into harmony with the habitual thinking. It is only a question of time. There is no guesswork about the processes. There is an absolutely inexorable law that *like must produce like.* Every thought that passes through our mind is a seed that we throw out into the soil, the world, and that must give a harvest like itself.

Even with the most positive thoughts a mind can imagine, external signs of the aging process are eminent. The role of a facial surgeon is to help the patient create a more youthful appearance than right thinking *alone* can achieve. When both parties are focused on the power of positive thought, results can be extraordinary.

As facial surgeons are able to envision the outcome of their surgery before the operation takes place, patients must have the capacity to envision themselves as younger, through and through, day by day, hour by hour. *Long-lasting results* are achieved when the patient's own thoughts are directed toward a youthful state of mind and the facial surgeon takes on the additional role of "life coach."

If you have colleagues or friends who are considering retirement, have them read this chapter. It could increase their career span beyond what they thought possible. Imagine how many more people could be helped, how many lives could be changed for the better. Imagine how much grander "the edifice" will become.

■ Reference

1. Marden, OS. Peace, Power, and Plenty. New York, NY: Thomas Crowell: 1909

10 The Vanity Factor

A common question that arises during the consultation with a prospective facial surgery patient is this: "Doctor, am I vain to consider having aesthetic surgery?" The following is a set of facts that the facial surgeon can use to offset those concerns.

The first order of business is to define the word *vanity*. I tell my patients that "vain" individuals are those who are so obsessed by their appearance that it interferes with their ability to function in society, those who cannot walk past a mirror or plate glass window without making sure everything is "just right."

I contrast such individuals with the example of people who exercise personal pride in their appearance, who bathe every day, shave accordingly, style and brush their hair, coordinate their clothes, use accessories appropriately, and pay attention to their posture and weight. There is nothing vain about these individuals, nothing vain about individuals who invest in themselves by putting their best face—their best *self*—forward, every day.

The *career enhancement factor* in looking one's best must not be understated. Among other things, I inform my facial surgery colleagues—and patients—about a July 2010 *Newsweek* survey[1] taken of hiring managers and job seekers. In the context of this book, prospective patients are hirers. The survey concluded that beauty (or handsomeness) *in the workplace* matters, that *it pays to look one's best.*

The following is extracted from an article written by Jessica Bennett about this survey.

> We've all heard the stories about how pretty people have it easy: babies smile more around good-looking parents; handsome kids get better grades and jobs, and earn more money; the list goes on. Still, we'd probably all like to think that we've earned our jobs on merit alone—and that, in this economy, it's our skill that will get us back in the game. But if you believe the results of two new *Newsweek* polls, you'd better think again—because in the current job market, paying attention to your looks isn't just about vanity, it's about economic survival. Job candidates have always been

counseled to dress up for interviews. But our surveys suggest managers are looking beyond wardrobe and evaluating how "physically attractive" applicants are. [How attractive (healthy) they are inside their skin, inside their skull. Facial surgeons should be aware that patients considering "hiring" us to perform surgery are sizing us up, as we are them.]

Newsweek conducted an online survey of 202 corporate hiring managers, from human-resource employees to senior-level VPs, as well as a telephone survey of a nationally representative sample of 964 members of the public, only to confirm what no qualified (or unqualified) employee wants to admit: that in all elements of the workplace, from hiring to politics to promotions, even, *looks matter,* and they matter hard.

The article goes on to list the eight most interesting revelations from the survey, which I summarize as follows:

1. *Looks matter at work.* Almost two-thirds of managers said they believed an *un*attractive (yet qualified) job candidate would have a harder time getting hired and believed that, once a person was hired, looks would continue to affect the way managers rated job performance.

2. *Looks matter more than education.* In a rating of nine character attributes, looks came in third, below experience and confidence, but above where a candidate went to school and a sense of humor. Does that mean candidates should throw away their college funds on cosmetic surgery? Probably not; but it does show that not all recruiters (patients) are looking for an Ivy League diploma.

3. *Put your money where your mouth is.* (We suppose that could be taken literally.) Sixty percent of hiring managers advised spending as much time and money on making sure applicants look attractive as on an impressive resume.

4. *It's more important for women.* As a whole, women were perceived to benefit more from their looks: almost 40% of managers believed that being "very good-looking" was more of an advantage for women than for men.

5. *Personnel directors discriminate against people who are overweight.* Almost 75% of Americans may be overweight, according to the U.S. Centers for Disease Control, yet the fact remains that humans discriminate against fat people at work and in life. Two-thirds of business managers said they believed some managers would hesitate before hiring a qualified job candidate who was significantly overweight.

6. *Managers also prefer young people* (or people who appear and act young). Of the managers surveyed, 84% said they believed some bosses would hesitate before hiring qualified job candidates who looked much older than the employees who would be their coworkers.

7. *Hiring is based on looks.* Two-thirds of hiring managers said they believed companies should be allowed to hire people based on looks when a job requires an employee to be the face of a company at retail stores or in sales.
8. *Confidence is important too!* Confidence and experience, of course, can still go a long way when it comes to succeeding at work. Remember, these ranked first and second on a list of the most important employee attributes.

The *Newsweek* survey is an indication that the future is bright for physicians who choose to specialize in aesthetic plastic surgery, that enhancing one's appearance tends to bolster every hiring factor that ranks above it. The following letter from a satisfied patient makes the point.

> Dear Dr. McCollough,
>
> The surgery you performed on me has truly had a positive influence on my life. As I have said on many occasions "face to riches," has been one of the very best decisions of my life.
>
> As you know I had a very bad accident which left me feeling my face and confidence were in bad condition 7 years ago. After talking to you, seeing your institute, meeting your team, and especially when you looked at me and said don't worry I'll take care of you, I was convinced to move forward and schedule my surgery.
>
> The road to recovery has been great. You have fulfilled your promise of taking care of me along with your other doctors, nurses, and staff. The positives in my life are enormous. I can breathe better, resulting in more restful sleep. Work business is up (while others complain they are down) compliments of my eyes (eyelids) and looks are coming my way again instilling confidence, and yes I've met a really great lady. My face is not perfect, which I did not want and you assured me you would not create a "new" face, just a better one.
>
> I just wanted to take time to thank you and your team for helping make all this possible.
>
> Sincerely,
>
> E. L.

The letter you've just read is what keeps me going to my clinic every day. It is what I hear as I talk with patients who have taken the initiative to enhance their appearance, and thus, their lives. Life is better, not only as a result of the surgical changes made in their external appearance, but by the image of themselves, seen by their mind's eye.

■ Reference

1. Bennett, Jessica (18 July 2010). "How much is beauty worth at work?" http://www. newsweek.com/poll-how-much-beauty-worth-work-74305, retrieved 31 July 2017

11 Skin and Beyond

The skin envelope is the largest organ of the human body. In that regard, it is also one of the earliest indicators that the biological systems that keep an individual "well" may be out of balance. This is a primary reason I routinely have prospective patients complete a medical questionnaire, undergo premedical testing, and obtain medical clearance from the patient's personal physician. As an appearance-enhancing surgeon, I want to know if a health problem exists. It helps me determine the nature and extent of the treatment I recommend for each patient and the facility in which it is to be performed.

Rather than simply treating *the visible* signs of aging, appearance-enhancement professionals in my institute provide skin condition assessments. They also provide therapies that are designed not only to make the skin *look* better, but also to help restore the skin after the ravages of aging and years of sun and wind exposure, from the inside out.

■ Nonsurgical Rejuvenation Procedures

A variety of procedures and products that camouflage the signs of aging are available. And the numbers grow with each passing year. Young facial surgeons can expect to be bombarded by sales representatives offering "the latest" technology or a machine/device that "every aesthetic surgeon must have in their practice.

My advice is to "go slowly." Think twice—and thrice—before purchasing or entering into a long-term lease for expensive equipment. Technology changes so rapidly that before the first machine is paid off, it is "out of style." Seek companies that will lease equipment—and in some cases, operators—*on a daily basis*. These companies will bring the equipment to your office on days you have patients scheduled and take the equipment away after the last patient is treated.

I have a standing practice of asking sales personnel to provide *histological proof* from independent researchers to verify claims made by the company selling a product, device, or piece of equipment. In too many cases, such evidence is not forthcoming. I interpret such *in*action as meaning *no evidence exists.*

In my mind, a facial surgeon's practice should be more than a drive-by filling station for commercially-created injectable fillers and muscle-paralyzing agents (neuromodulators). It should be an age and appearance management center—one firmly rooted in evidence-based medicine and surgery.

Clearly, advanced skin care programs and products can give one's skin a more youthful appearance. Medical-grade, injectable fillers provide *temporary* improvement in wrinkles and hollowed areas caused by aging, but many clients are looking for more. They want *to be* as healthy as they look and look as healthy as they are. And they want these things longer than some of the temporary therapies can provide. More importantly, patients deserve to know the pros and cons of temporary therapies, as compared with more permanent alternatives. As part of a physician's "informed consent" regarding treatment, the alternatives should be discussed prior to treatment.

When more permanent eradication of the undesirable signs of volume loss is desired, the *patient's own collagen* can be transplanted through tiny incisions by a facial surgeon duly trained in the technique (**Fig. 11.1**).

Neurotoxins minimize the kinds of wrinkling and scowls that occur with *exaggerated* facial expressions, but not those when a face is "at rest." Demonstrating this to a patient in front of a mirror will help prevent having an

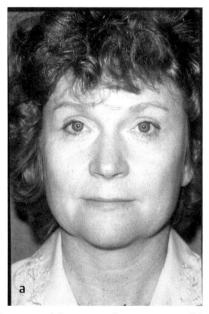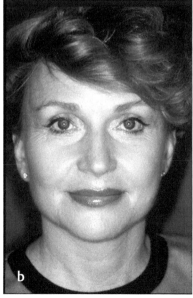

Fig. 11.1 **(a)** Prior to collagen injection. **(b)** After collagen injection.

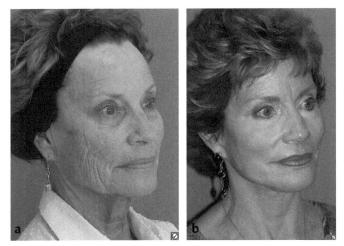

Fig. 11.2   **(a)** Prior to face lift and skin resurfacing. **(b)** After facelifting and full face skin resurfacing.

ill-informed and dissatisfied patient. Patients should know that—for best results—retreatment every several months is required.

Level I laser therapy and superficial skin polishing (microdermabrasion) are provided by many aesthetic physicians and surgeons. These procedures remove the dull, scaly skin that collects on the surface as new skin is created underneath, giving one's skin a younger, healthier glow and smoother texture for a short period of time. For *level II and III* conditions more surgically oriented therapies are required, procedures that can provide results that last in terms of years (**Fig. 11.2**).

■ Skin Polishing Products

A wide variety of commercial skin care products are available on over-the-counter, mail-order, and television commercial markets. Simply stated, some of them are more *hype* than *help*. Some misleadingly represent themselves as "facelifts in a bottle." While the term *facelift* is loosely applied to upgrading any edifice, it is a stretch to call the skin polishing effects of topically applied commercial products a facelift (**Fig. 11.3**).

Among the menagerie of available products, a select few have been determined (through research and experience) to be helpful in giving the skin a more youthful appearance. It is a scientific fact that products that require *a prescription* from a physician—and that are administered under the oversight of a physician—tend to be more effective. The reason is that the concentration and combinations of active ingredients of physician-monitored products are

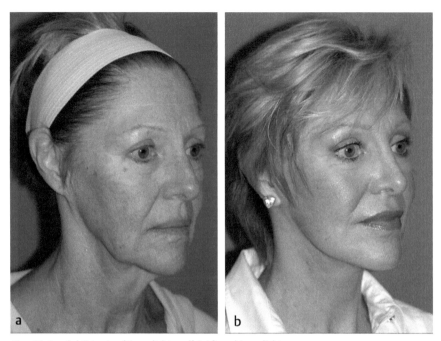

Fig. 11.3 **(a)** Prior to skin polishing. **(b)** After skin polishing.

manufactured to higher specifications and must meet stringent health and safety guidelines. However, it is important to note that just because a physician endorses a product or procedure, it does not mean that the product has been subjected to scientific scrutiny. It is a sad state of affairs, but many physician spokespersons are compensated actors or salespersons who just happen to have medical degrees.

It is important that facial surgeons and aestheticians alike realize—and communicate to their patients/clients—that the vast majority of *nonsurgical* rejuvenation therapies are designed to produce *temporary results*. Longer-lasting results—and lasting provider-client relationships—are realized when patients are duly informed about the cost/benefit ratio of products and procedures recommended. Patients also benefit when the skin care professionals providing *nonsurgical* procedures and products work hand in hand with facial surgeons, and vice versa.

■ The Skin as an Indicator of Health or Illness

Facial surgeons must never lose sight of the fact that they are, first, physicians/ scientists sworn to the Hippocratic Oath. The tenet "First, do no harm" should be at the forefront of a surgeon's decision-making process. The patient's health and well-being must be the first—and final—consideration.

Human skin is an indicator of conditions that exist beneath it. Undiagnosed medical conditions (hormone imbalances, thyroid deficiencies, collagen disorders, poor nutrition, stress, etc.) are often reflected in the appearance and texture of one's skin. It is for this reason that a physician should be involved with any "skin care center" or "spa."

Skin care, nutrition, and weight and age management should be approached from both directions: *inside out* and *outside in*. In that respect the skin should be viewed as a two-way mirror.

From a blood sample, a facial surgeon can determine whether a prospective patient's hormones are out of balance, whether the patient needs to supplement their diet, or whether indicators of biological imbalance of the patient's internal organ systems exist. If it is determined that imbalance is present, a rejuvenation specialist can recommend the appropriate corrective measures prior to undertaking a surgical procedure requiring optimal healing. In some cases, referral to the patient's personal physician or a medical specialist is indicated.

It is virtually impossible to separate an individual's appearance from their health. Over the years, I have found that *patients who do the things that are required to look their best tend to find better health*, even if finding better health was not their primary objective when consulting me.

■ Weight Management: Its Effect on Skin, Health, Aging, and Facial Features

It should come as no surprise that as an individual gains weight, the skin surrounding the face and body substructures is stretched, making those structures even more susceptible to premature sags and bulges, especially if the individual loses large amounts of weight. Roller-coaster weight swings can be even more damaging. Each time the skin is stretched, elasticity is lost. The process leads to sags and droops throughout the entire body. This fundamental—and documentable—characteristic of the skin of mammals lies at the heart of using "tissue expanders" or "serial excisions" in reconstructive surgery.

During consultation, I am often asked if weight gain or loss will affect the treatment plan I recommend. My answer to patients is this: *"A 10- to 12-pound weight swing will make very little difference.* If you plan to lose more than that, let's wait until you get to within that 10 to 12 pounds of what you think your *realistic weight* will be."

I emphasize the word *realistic* because most people have both an "ideal weight" *and* a "realistic weight" (one they are able to maintain). I also tell patients that it is fruitless to lose beyond their "realistic weight," knowing that they are likely to gain it back.

Another fundamental principle of nutrition and health applies here. When a body is losing weight, it is in a *catabolic* state, that is, it is cannibalizing itself through a process known to biochemists as "negative nitrogen balance." First stored carbohydrates are cannibalized, then fat, and finally, muscle. I recommend that any patient engaged in a weight reduction program reverse the process to an *anabolic* state (positive nitrogen balance) prior to undergoing surgery. It is my hypothesis that not doing so is why patients undergoing surgical procedures following massive weight loss do not heal as well as other patients.

I also explain that managing one's weight is not nearly as complicated as one might think. It is a matter of self-discipline and keeping score—balancing the number and kind of calories ingested each day with the number of calories expended while one goes about one's daily routine. Clearly, more physical activity burns more calories. But exercise alone *has not* proven to be the answer to weight management. For example, one must walk a mile (at a rapid pace) to burn off the number of calories that one takes in with two cookies, a nondietetic drink, or a small piece of cake or pie.

I now share with you the conversation I have with my patients who are serious about losing weight. Most commercial "diet" plans are *product (and profit) driven*. The client is expected to purchase the meals produced by the company.

In truth, a bit of nutritional education allows clients/patients to do their own shopping and meal planning, at great savings.

Here are the simple facts. If one *eliminates* just 100 calories per day (by avoidance or through exercise), at the end of only 30 days, 3,000 calories will have been eliminated from the system. That is the number of calories required to create (or burn) *1 pound of fat*. Simply stated, if people consistently eliminate just 100 calories per day from their food and drink intake, at the end of a year, they will have lost 12 pounds. Conversely, if they consistently *add* the equivalent of 100 calories per day to their diet, 12 pounds of fat will accumulate in 12 months. This simple mathematical equation is the "secret" to weight management. Still, many patients need encouragement. There can be no better encouragement than from a surgeon in whom the patient has full confidence, the kind of confidence created during the initial visit/consultation of a doctor-patient relationship grounded in trust, a trust that is never violated, or taken for granted.

■ Treatment and Product Options for Creating More Youthful Skin

The skin of the face is the draping under which the skeletal, muscular, and adipose architecture exists. It is also the focus of skin resurfacing procedures (laser therapy, chemical peels, and dermabrasions) that provide a more youthful, vibrant external appearance. In the hands of a well-trained facial surgeon, each of these skin resurfacing modalities is effective. What *is not equal* is the expense factor in providing chemical peeling, dermabrasion, or laser therapies to the skin. The cost (to the physician) of the supplies and chemicals of a peel is usually less than $100 for a dozen or more cases. The cost to purchase a level II and III dermabrasion machine and abrasive brushes is in the range of $2,000. The cost to purchase a laser can range from $35,000 to more than $100,000. The life span of a level II or III chemical peeling formula is a lifetime. The life span of a dermabrasion unit and brushes is a decade. The life span of the most expensive treatment modality (a laser machine) is 5 to 7 years. The surgeon should also explore the cost of maintaining a laser over that span of time. I once heard a colleague say to an auditorium full of colleagues, "Before I came to this meeting, I visited one of the storage rooms in my office. I did a quick survey and determined that I had approximately *a million dollars' worth* of outdated lasers and noninvasive equipment doing nothing but collecting dust in that room."

With the appropriate training and experience, a facial surgeon can achieve the same—or very similar—results with any of the three methods of skin resurfacing. The message from a colleague who has tried and tested each skin resurfacing modality is this: Do the math. Obtain the training. Deliver more, for less.

■ Smart Nutrition: Feeding the Skin and Its Contents

As a biological organ, the skin of a human being relies upon proper nutrition—and all factors related to the metabolism of each ingested building block—to produce youthful, healthy cells during each phase of the process that many of us learned about in high school biology called "mitosis," or "cell division."

As is the case with a maturing baby, if deprived of essential foods, vitamins, and minerals, the baby fails to develop properly. In that respect, each new cell *of the skin* is a "baby" cell and must be nourished accordingly.

However, the only way that one will ever know if the cells of the body are being properly nourished is through scientific testing. From a single blood sample, virtually every vitamin, mineral, and amino acid (the building blocks of collagen production) can be measured. When the cellular levels of these nutritional elements are found to be deficient, the right combination—and amounts—of the missing parts can be provided with pharmaceutical-grade supplements. Simply stated, there is no other way to really know if patients need nutritional supplements or if they are taking the right combinations or doses. And the facial surgeon who understands—and provides—this holistic approach to skin health distinguishes themself from the competition.

■ Hormone Balancing for Women and Men

Earlier I said that facial surgeons must think of themselves—and recommend treatment—first as a physician, to whom their patients entrust their care.

There is no debate among health care professionals that hormone levels drop with every year past the age of 30. In women, the process happens rapidly, causing obvious changes in the way a woman feels and looks—a condition known as menopause.

In men, the process is known as andropause, and it occurs more gradually—often sparing men the flash sweats, mood swings, and fluid retention. However, by the age of 50, both men and women experience measurable drops in the hormones that sustained a youthful appearance and heightened performance and positive outlooks on life. And making sure that the patient's hormonal system is "in balance" lets the patient know that a facial surgeon will do everything possible to enhance the health and appearance of every individual who entrusts their care to that surgeon. It is the demonstration of such a commitment that solidifies the long-term doctor-patient relationship this book emphasizes. In addition, a healthy hormonal system enhances the work performed by a facial surgeon, and the way a patient feels.

In today's complex, highly regulated—and highly publicized—medical environment, going above and beyond what is generally expected is the exception rather than the rule. There is no reason why holistic-minded facial surgeons cannot create a new "normal," at least within their practice setting. Not only does a facial surgeon have the opportunity to do so, but the fact that the opportunity exists could raise it to the level of a responsibility.

■ The Stress Factor: Speeding Up the Aging Process and How to Slow It Down

Every year, scientists learn more about the aging process in human beings. And while no one has, yet, discovered how to arrest it, ways to speed it up are well known. The mind-body factor was discussed in Chapter 8. The secret lies in the mind of the only species on Earth awarded "free will" at the time of its creation. A little-recognized element of the gift known as free will is that different people respond to the alternatives laid in their paths in different ways.

As both James Allen and Dr. Orison Marden pointed out, it is *how* one responds to pressing circumstances that determines those circumstances' effects on the body, and on the mind. Some people absorb stress as a sponge takes on water. Others shed it as Teflon sheds water. The "sponges" of the world are much more apt to experience the physical and mental effects of stress than "Teflon people." Facial surgeons are more likely to see the sponges seeking their services and being willing to deal with their reasons for requesting surgical intervention.

Stress may be one of the most manageable enemies to longevity, productivity, and happiness. That having been said, *stress relief* may be one of the ways to arrest many of the unwanted signs and symptoms of aging. That is why, in my patient information book, I include a chapter on stress, grief, and loss management.

The holistic-minded, patient-oriented facial surgeon is both able and willing to share these fundamental truths with patients. A period of aerobic exercise, relaxation, or meditation is one way to "let go" of pent-up stress. A professionally administered "therapeutic facial" or massage relaxes muscles, lowers tension levels, and creates the release of the body's own natural chemical relaxants and painkillers (endorphins.) This—coupled with reflexology therapy and a peaceful, professional environment—allows one to let go of the kinds of tension that promote premature aging and interfere with productivity in the workplace.

When the pressures of stress or the weight of grief becomes too heavy to manage with the aforementioned therapies, facial surgeons who have developed the kind of relationship with their patients that this book advocates are in a position to recommend the services of a licensed counselor or therapist. They are able to explain to their patient that asking for help under these circumstances *is not* a sign of weakness, but a demonstration of wisdom.

Imagine the possibilities when facial surgery is viewed—not as a procedure-driven profession—but as a specialty that *expects* its practitioners to invigorate and enhance their patient's mind, face, body, and soul.

This truth is what attracted me to aesthetic and reconstructive surgery. Witnessing theory become reality on a daily basis in my practice is what keeps me coming to work at the age of 73. It is why, as long as I am competent, I have no plans to do anything else. Why would I? What other activity could give one so much pleasure? So much fulfillment? So many opportunities to help fellow human beings make the most of every day—every year—they live? And after all, is this not what being a "doctor" is all about?

■ An Example of Tilting the Scales of Opportunity

The following letter was received from a patient (**Fig. 11.4**) on October 19, 2000:

Dear Dr. McCollough,

I just wanted to thank you and your staff for the wonderful care and treatment you've given me. My facial surgery of my nose and chin is exactly what I wanted, and the results are actually so much better than I had expected.

I didn't realize how this would change my life so positively. I find with all the compliments I've received, I've started holding my head up more and making more eye contact with others. I believe this gives me more confidence and the appearance of having more confidence. In turn, I have been entrusted with more meaningful work projects and had more opportunities for success in my career.

I can never thank you enough. I will always remember the kindness of you and your staff, which made my experience with this surgery so delightful. I would be happy to share my experience with any of the prospective patients. Thank you again so much.

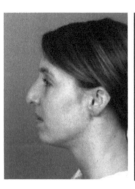 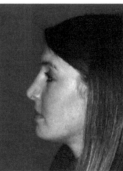

Fig. 11.4   (a) Before and **(b)** after photos of a grateful facial surgery patient.

II Procedures That Comprise a Facial Surgery Practice

12 Nasal Plastic Surgery: Rhinoplasty

Rhinoplasty is the most difficult facial surgical procedure to master. It requires the ability to apply—in the operating room—principles rooted in the aesthetic arts as well as Newtonian laws (physics and structural engineering).

Most rhinoplasties are performed because the patient desires an improvement in appearance and/or nasal function. The patient may simply want a nose that is in harmony with the rest of the face rather than one that is out of proportion with respect to the other facial features (**Fig. 12.1**). On the other hand, it may be that the nose has been injured and is becoming progressively more disfigured the older the patient becomes.

At times patients have deformities of the inside of the nose that impair breathing or *contribute to headaches* or to sinus disease. These problems cannot be satisfactorily treated medically without simultaneously straightening the external nose.

Like faces, every nose is different; some noses are too long, some are too wide, some have large humps, some project away from the face, and so on.

A facial surgeon should strive to make each patient's nose fit the rest of the face. If a surgeon was not properly trained to perform rhinoplasty *and septoplasty*, that surgeon should refer the patient to a colleague who specializes in the procedures.

The alterations recommended by a facial surgeon should be determined by many factors, including the patient's height, age, skin thickness, and ethnic

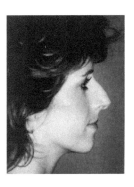 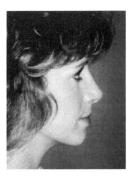

Fig. 12.1 A nose that is too large is "out of proportion" to the other facial features. Reducing its size and altering its shape brings it into harmony and enhances the other facial features.

background and the configuration of other features such as the forehead, eyes, and chin. In short, the objective should be to achieve a *natural-looking nose* rather than one that appears to have been created by a surgeon.

In its simplest form, a well-conceived rhinoplasty is one in which anatomical structures that are in excess are removed or reduced, those that are deficient are augmented, and those that need no alteration are undisturbed.

I have published numerous articles (and a textbook[1]) on rhinoplasty. Each focuses on the intricacies of the procedure—specific aesthetic and functional techniques to accomplish the most "ideal" nose for a given patient. I have organized and conducted numerous continuing education seminars on rhinoplasty. Each one has dealt with preoperative assessment, surgical techniques, and postoperative management. Each has emphasized that there is no one-size-fits-all technique for any phase of the rhinoplasty operation. Rather it is a condition-specific exercise in surgical judgment and dexterity.

I do not subscribe to the ideology that every nose should be taken apart and reconstructed with grafts. Clearly, there are noses that require major reconstruction—those that have been mutilated by multiple surgeries or major trauma.

To date, I have performed nearly 6,000 rhinoplasties. As the numbers began to mount, I found myself removing less cartilage, especially in the nasal tip. The undesirable effects of aggressive removal of tip cartilage may not appear until 20 years have passed, but they are certain to appear.

In recent years, I have focused more on reshaping tip cartilages with sutures (similar to the technique described in my 1981 article "Systematic Approach to Correction of the Nasal Tip in Rhinoplasty[2]." With additional experience and long-term follow-up, I have modified the technique since the original article was published. I recommend suture modification of tip cartilages, using sutures that dissolve within 6 to 8 weeks, when necessary. Permanent sutures are not necessary. After that time, the tissues will maintain the shape initially created by suturing.

The intent of this discussion on rhinoplasty is not to describe a step-by-step methodology. That is available in my book *Nasal Plastic Surgery*.[1] Here, I wish to emphasize a *condition-specific process of thought* and several teaching points that led me to this way of thinking. The process is an algorithmic surgical progression derived from Ockham's (razor) logic—*when many options are possible, the simplest one is generally the correct one.* This line of thinking will avoid disastrous outcomes and shorten the rhinoplasty "learning curve" for facial surgery colleagues. That same logic should be applied to the procedures discussed in the following chapters.

■ At What Age Can Rhinoplasty Be Performed?

An often asked question is at what age nasal plastic and reconstructive surgery can be performed. If a severe breathing problem (or headache issue) is present, even in a child, the anatomical obstruction should be conservatively corrected. With children, additional surgery at "maturity" may be required to obtain the optimal result. Certain limitations exist in children that preclude performing the definitive correction prior to puberty. Disturbing "growth centers" in the nose prior to maturity is thought to arrest nasal development.

Ordinarily, girls are mature enough to undergo rhinoplasty by the age of 15 (boys by age 17). However, I find it necessary to individualize this factor because some boys and girls mature at earlier ages. So that I can monitor their growth and maturation, I prefer to see these young men and women *at whatever age* they become interested in having a rhinoplasty, even though surgical correction may be delayed.

Early correction of unwanted nasal deformities can often give young people more self-confidence and improved self-esteem. *A parent or guardian should always come with a minor to the consultation visit.*

At the opposite end of the spectrum, approximately 30% of the rhinoplasties I perform are on patients over the age of 40. Many older patients remark that they have disliked their noses "all their life" and have now decided to have corrective surgery. Providing the patient is in good health, *it is never too late in life to have a rhinoplasty.* It is often performed as part of a facial rejuvenation program (along with facelift and eyelid plastic surgery) to improve the undesirable signs of aging.

A longer drooping nose may be a "telltale" sign of aging, and repositioning of the drooping tip of the nose can be performed to give a more youthful appearance (**Fig. 12.2**).

Whenever a nasal airway problem is identified, the appropriate "functional" procedures are performed at the same sitting.

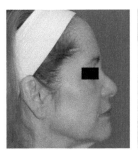 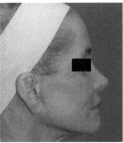

Fig. 12.2 With aging, the tip of the nose becomes longer due to loss of the tip support.

A little-appreciated cause of headaches is a *septal deviation* that impacts the membranes of nasal turbinates. In many cases a "spur" (sharp edge) can be identified at a point where an old fracture occurred. Relieving this impaction can often eliminate headaches—or at least reduce their frequency and severity. It is a predictable—and often unappreciated—treatment of headaches.

A helpful presurgery test for patients who suffer from headaches and are found to have septal deformities during examination is to have the patient spray the nose with a decongesting nasal spray at the first sign of a headache to shrink the membranes and, temporarily, relieve the pressure exerted by the spur. If the spray aborts the headache, it is likely that a functional septoplasty will provide long-term relief.

I share a statement that I have found to be extremely helpful when dealing with revisional or posttraumatic noses, including the preempting sentence. I say to the patient, "Now, I must tell you the last thing you want to hear. Noses that are crooked, have been severely injured, or have undergone previous surgery are more difficult to correct, *and may require more than one procedure*."

I often consult with patients who have undergone multiple previous surgeries and are still left with aesthetic and functional issues. Missing structural components and scarring create challenges to the revisional rhinoplastic surgeon, thereby introducing more variables in the outcome. Sometimes, cartilage and bone grafts used to reconstruct nasal structures simply do not survive transfer. Existing scarring makes dissection difficult and skin malleability unpredictable. Postoperative, intralesional steroids (usually triamcinolone 7–10 mg/mL in combination with dilute 5-fluorouracil injected at 3-week intervals after surgery) can prevent the reaccumulation of postoperative scarring—especially in the supratip region.

■ The Planning Process

Prior to rhinoplasty, photographs are taken so that the characteristics of the nose and face can be studied, documented, and shared with the patient. The operation is planned in much the same way an architect plans a house; the goal is not only to improve the shape of the nose but also to bring it into harmony with the entire face. Leonardo da Vinci's facial proportions are used to create the aesthetic/cosmetic portions of the treatment plan (**Fig. 12.3**).

For patients who live far away, a teleconference/photographic analysis and interview can be performed prior to an in-office consultation, thereby shortening the time from the first call to the operation. For medicolegal purposes, it is necessary to explain that final recommendations will be provided at the time of a face-to-face consultation.

As mentioned in Chapter 10, many patients who present to facial surgeons have deep-seated feelings of insecurity that are related to the appearance of one

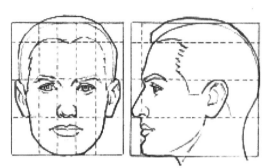

Fig. 12.3 The "ideal" facial proportions are demonstrated in this diagram. The nose should fit into the middle one-third of the face, as depicted here. From a profile view, the chin should be in line with the lower lip.

or more features of their face. These patients require extraordinary attention. It takes more than surgical alterations of anatomical features in the operating room to help them "heal" from years of insecurity. Enhancing a patient's self-esteem requires a genuine interest *in the individual,* professionally expressed at the time of consultation, and throughout the healing process.

The value of the facial surgeon's staff cannot be overstated. Heartfelt compliments offered to patients by every staff member—at every encounter—build self-esteem. Patients seem to appreciate inquiries about how family, friends, coworkers, or fellow students are responding to their "new look." If there is a secret to treating the psychological aspect of changing the size and shape of a patient's nose, it lies with these words: *ongoing positive reinforcement, provided at every opportunity.*

But what if the operation did not rise to the expectations of the patient, or the surgeon? My advice—and practice—in such cases is to be honest. *Admit that there is a residual problem.* Stress the need to allow the nose to heal (for *at least* 9–12 months) and then reassess the situation. However, have the patient return at 1- to 2-month intervals to evaluate the healing process. Take photographs to document the changes taking place as the nose heals.

If after a year from the time of the original operation, the surgeon feels qualified to correct the problem—*correct the problem!* On the other hand, if the surgeon does not feel qualified to correct remaining issues, that surgeon should refer the patient to a colleague experienced in revisional rhinoplasty. The absolutely improper way to manage an unsatisfactory result is to ignore it, or deny that it exists. Patients are smart. They recognize the fact that doctors aren't perfect and respect an honest admission that the operation did not meet the expectations. So do juries in courts of law.

The following is an unsolicited letter received from a happy rhinoplasty patient. I share it here to demonstrate the opportunity given to facial surgeons to change the lives—in a positive way—of the patients for whom we care.

■ A Life-Changing Testimonial

Dr. McCollough,

I wanted to personally thank you again for the life-changing effect you have had on my life. In July 2005 I came to your office feeling very insecure about the way I looked, but you, like my family, saw through to the vibrant young woman inside.

I remember talking to you about what I expected and you were thrilled that I was not interested in having a "tiny pug nose" but that I wanted a more elegant and refined version of myself. That is precisely what you gave me.

Before my rhinoplasty, I was always cautious about the way I positioned myself in a room, making sure that no one ever caught a glimpse of my profile.

I was a freshman in college and didn't involve myself in many on-campus activities because having to constantly be aware of my nose was exhausting. I didn't date many guys but instead stayed with the same dead end comfort zone that I had been in for the last 4 years.

Don't get me wrong, I would still go places and move toward my goal of attending dental school; I just wasn't having much fun doing it.

I am happy to report that following my surgery I rushed for . . . sorority and graduated with honors from the University of . . . I gained many friends and was involved in many on-campus clubs and intramural activities. Whereas before, I always felt timid when working with patients, following the surgery I got a job in a dental clinic which helped prepare me for where I am today.

I am now attending the University of . . . College of Dentistry. I will be graduating in the spring of 2013, and I love what I'm doing.

Since last seeing you, I have also met the man of my dreams and we are getting married in March 2011.

One thing I look forward to is basking in the joy of that day and not having to worry about the angle that the pictures are taken in or who is looking at my nose instead of at me. I am sure you get these letters every day, but I wanted to thank you. I have always been this girl, but you gave me the courage to show her to the world.

I sincerely thank you,

S. H.

While I have received numerous letters and personal testimonials of a similar nature, each one underscores the opportunity—and responsibility—a facial plastic surgeon is given to impact the lives of fellow human beings, to open gateways "to the world" that otherwise would have remained closed. I can't imagine spending my life doing anything else.

■ References

1. McCollough EG Nasal Plastic Surgery. Philadelphia, PA: W. B. Saunders;1994
2. "Systematic Approach to Correcting the Nasal Tip in Rhinoplasty", McCollough E.G.; Mangat, D. Arch Otolaryngol 1981;107(1):12–16

13 Chin Augmentation

It is often necessary to recommend surgery for a receding chin, either in connection with a *rhinoplasty, a facelift, or liposuction, or as an isolated procedure.* The chin is an important feature in creating comprehensive facial harmony.

When facial plastic surgeons examine a patient's profile, they look to see if the chin projection approaches a line dropped vertically from the lower lip, as Renaissance genius Leonardo da Vinci concluded it should (**Fig. 13.1**).

A small chin is a feminine characteristic. A strong chin is a masculine characteristic. In women, I generally choose an implant that *slightly* undercorrects a receding chin. In a man, an implant that brings the chin into alignment with the vertical line extending from the lower lip is preferred.

Too much recession of the chin, particularly when accompanied by a slanting forehead, will cause the features to taper to a point in the midface, rather than give the vertical alignment described by da Vinci.

A discerning facial surgeon may actually advise against other facial procedures unless the projection of the chin can be brought into balance.

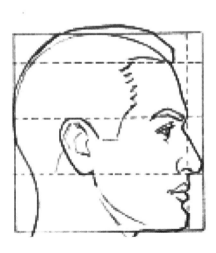

Fig. 13.1 From the profile, the chin alignment should approximate a line extended vertically from the lower lip.

Of course there are patients who desire chin augmentation alone. Many patients who choose to undergo face and neck lifts (and who have a receding chin accompanied by excess fatty tissue underneath) can achieve a more aesthetically pleasing profile by having a chin implant and submental liposuction performed in conjunction with their face and neck lifts (**Fig. 13.2**).

While I have performed chin augmentation through a variety of methods, I generally prefer an *intraoral* approach. The procedure is performed through an incision several millimeters superior to the crease between the lower lip and gum. A fatal error is to make the incision directly into the gingival–labial sulcus. Doing so makes creating a liquid-proof closure virtually impossible and increases the risk of postoperative infection.

Absorbable sutures are used to close the intraoral wound—first the muscular layers, then mucous membranes. When the scar in the mucous membrane "matures," it is well camouflaged. Most patients may resume their preoperative activities within about 1 week.

"Twilight" anesthesia (conscious sedation) is used for chin augmentation.

For more than 4 decades, a condition-specific, individually created, medical-grade mesh has been my implant of choice. It is placed *beneath the periosteum* and increases chin projection by supporting the soft tissues overlying the gonion of the mandible, or jawbone.

Chin augmentation is based upon the same concept as breast augmentation (mammoplasty), wherein an implant is placed under the soft tissue. In the chin operation, the implant is placed (subperiosteally) on top of the mandible so that the soft tissues (skin, fat, and muscles) rest upon the implant, rather than on the bone (**Fig. 13.3**).

In 4 decades of using soft, medical-grade mesh implants, I am not aware of a single case of bone absorption deep to the implant—a sequela often seen with hard silastic implants.

Medical-grade materials are sometimes employed to make artificial heart components or arteries, for reconstruction about the eye and nose, to repair

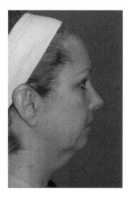 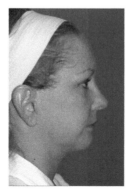

Fig. 13.2 When the chin recedes behind an imaginary line dropped vertically from the lower lip, an augmentation mentoplasty (chin implant) can correct the deficiency and provide facial harmony. This patient also had a cheek/neck facelift with liposuction at the jowls and neck.

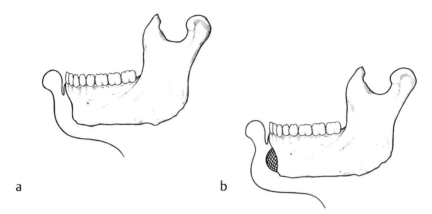

Fig. 13.3   **(a)** A receding chin is usually the result of a short mandible (jawbone). **(b)** An implant placed on the mandible supports the tissues, bringing the chin into better alignment.

hernias, and for many other purposes in various parts of the body. The material has been used in hundreds of cases and has a high record of safety and satisfaction. After a short time has elapsed, a mesh implant becomes practically the same consistency as the surrounding tissues and becomes incorporated into them. As is sometimes recommended for patients who have been diagnosed with mitral valve prolapse, I recommend that patients in whom any alloplastic implant has been placed, be placed on prophylactic antibiotic therapy.

In my mind, there are other advantages in using mesh or porous foam implants. The implant can be saturated with a broad-spectrum antibiotic solution prior to insertion.

Another advantage of a mesh or foam implant is tissue ingrowth. The patient's own collagen grows into the implant to help stabilize it.

Here is a good opportunity to share a key teaching point that applies *to all* implants, regardless of the material from which they are manufactured and the location in the body in which they are inserted. *No member of the operating team handles an implant with gloves that have touched the patient.* Doing so transfers microorganisms from the patient's skin to the surgeon's gloves, and then to the implant. In short, an implant touched with gloves that have come in contact with the patient's skin is a contaminated implant. And postoperative infection is more likely.

In my practice, patients receiving implants are treated—for 2 weeks—with prophylactic broad-spectrum antibiotics. In fact, almost all of my patients are, regardless of the procedures performed. Nonimplant patients receive antibiotics for 1 week. Patients who have undergone implant surgery receive them for an additional week.

Another point to remember is this: if an antibiotic is not circulating throughout the patient's bloodstream *when the surgical incision is made*, it is not considered a "prophylactic" antibiotic, but rather a "therapeutic" antibiotic.

14 Cheek/Malar Augmentation

In my practice, cheek implants (**Fig. 14.1**) are rarely indicated. Particularly as the procedure applies to the malar mound, I find it rarely necessary in facelift surgery. Rather, I have found that *repositioning/uplifting* tissues (that once covered the malar prominence and have descended because of aging) by performing a cheek lift creates the aesthetic enhancement that most patients require (see Chapter 20 on facelift surgery).

At the time of this writing, I am not a strong advocate of temporary fillers or fat grafting for this region, *if the patient is amenable to surgery*. I prefer to "volumize" the region by replacing the fat/soft tissue mound to its original position with a cheek lift procedure. I have found this practice not only to be more effective, but also to be the most predictable and economical method of re-creating a youthful "midface" (**Fig. 14.2**).

When a malar implant is advised, I generally prefer the "anatomical" silastic model, inserted through an intraoral incision made *vertically* at the gingival–mucosal sulcus, superior to the canine (cuspid) teeth. It is the incision preferred when open maxillary sinus antrostomy is performed. The implant is inserted using the same "no-touch" technique described with chin implants in a

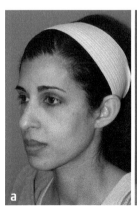 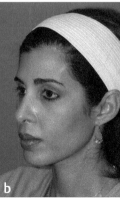

Fig. 14.1 (a) Before and **(b)** after photos of a patient who underwent cheek/malar augmentation with silastic implants.

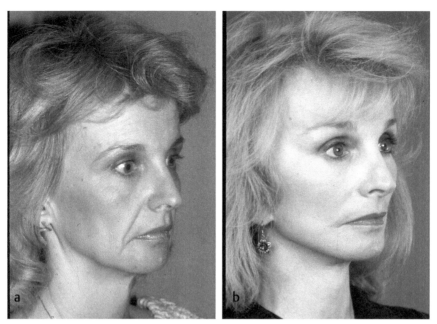

Fig. 14.2 **(a)** Before and **(b)** after photos of a patient who underwent a cheek lift with repositioning of sagging cheek tissues. No implant or injectable materials were used.

*sub*periosteal fashion, after a "made-to-size" pocket is created. The incision site is closed with an absorbable suture (usually chromic catgut.)

As is the case with all implant patients, prophylactic antibiotics are prescribed, for 2 weeks.

15 Lip Enhancement: Lifting and Augmentation

In the 21st century people from many ethnic backgrounds are becoming interested in having fuller, more youthful-looking lips. Injectable materials may provide temporary enhancement (see Chapter 25); however, I prefer methods that provide longer-term improvement. And although surgical correction might not be recommended for every patient, a surgical *lip lift* or an autologous augmentation graft using a patient's own fat and/or collagen can offer more permanent improvement to patients concerned about thin or aging lips (**Fig. 15.1**).

The *lip lift* is performed by excising a strip of skin above the top lip and below the bottom lip, then advancing the mucosal portion of the lips into the defect. I do not recommend this procedure in men, in whom a non-hair-bearing area just outside the vermilion border exists. The standard lip lift excises this non-hair-bearing area and causes the beard to crowd the vermilion, thereby creating a nonanatomical condition.

The key to lip line advancement lies in where and how the incisions are made and closed. Incisions beveled *away* from the midline of the vermilion line are recommended. Fine, delicate sutures, placed while using magnification, allow the facial surgeon to accurately approximate and evert the wound edges. Vertical mattress sutures placed at the Cupid's bow region are crucial to wound closure for thread-thin postsurgical scars. A running subcuticular, monofilament suture is preferred in other areas of the upper and lower lip.

For patients over 40, surgical lip enhancement is often combined with *skin resurfacing* (laser, chemical peel, or dermabrasion), certainly when rhytids are present. Because—more often than not—injecting "fillers" underneath the skin above the vermilion borders results in "duck lips," I do not recommend filling these regions.

In younger patients, lips may be enlarged by fat/fascia transplantation alone. In these cases, fascia can be harvested from the postauricular sulcus and overlying fascia of the postauricular musculature. Patients who have undergone previous facelift surgery have a sheet of favorable scar just beneath the subcutaneous tissue behind the ear. Mature scar is the ideal graft for lips, melolabial grooves, and deep glabellar creases.

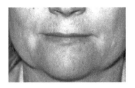 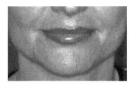

Fig. 15.1 (a) Prior to lip enhancement. **(b)** After lip enhancement.

With these new modifications in the technique, lip augmentation has become a popular procedure; and it can be performed with a high degree of satisfaction in men and women. Because full lips are a feminine characteristic, conservatism should be exercised in male patients.

In both men and women, aesthetic balance is the key. Lips that are too large create an unsightly condition. And in keeping with da Vinci's criteria for facial harmony, the lower lip should always be larger than the upper lip, by about 20%.

Grafting material is readily available when a superficial musculoaponeurotic system (SMAS)–imbricating facelift is performed. A continuous strip of the excised fat and SMAS overlying the parotid gland makes an ideal graft. In years past, a single graft was threaded in a tunnel made from one oral commissure to the other. In many cases the graft would twist, thereby creating a narrowing at the point of twisting during insertion. I corrected this tendency by creating two separate grafts (in both the upper and lower lip) anatomically joined in the midline through a separate incision. An additional advantage of this modification is that the grafts can be slightly overlapped to create a natural tubercle in the midline of the upper lip. This anatomical feature is not present in the aesthetically balanced lower lip.

Surgical incisions made for insertion of these grafts are closed with absorbable sutures, which usually dissolve within 5 to 7 days. The incision lines progress through the usual maturation process, in which the scar is discolored and lumpy for a few weeks. Eventually it blends into the surrounding tissues as it flattens and color differences disappear. But, as is the case with all scars, time is the friend of the surgeon.

Some patients may desire correction of the upper (or lower) lip only. Most patients, however, choose to have both done.

The mucosa proximal to the "wet line" of the lip will generally be advanced to the outside of the mouth. It takes several weeks for the "wet" mucosa to acclimate to its new environment outside the mouth. Copious amounts of lip moisturizers are required until this adaptation process takes place.

Either of the lip procedures can be performed as an isolated procedure or may be combined with other facial plastic surgical operations discussed in this book.

Patients should be told to expect the lips to be quite swollen after surgery. For several weeks they will appear "overcorrected." The rule of thumb that applies to *all surgical areas* should be shared with these patients: Swelling increases for the first 2 to 3 days after *any* procedure. Not much happens for the next

2 to 3 days. Then, on day 4 or 5, the swelling and bruising begin to subside. As a rule 80% of the maximum swelling that was present in the first few days subsides in 2 weeks; 90% subsides in 2 months. The remaining 10% goes away gradually over the ensuing months.

The preceding information will go a long way toward allaying a patient's anxiety and should be shared with the patient prior to surgery.

16 Otoplasty: Surgery for Protruding Ears

Large protruding ears often cause deeper emotional upset than is generally realized by the patient's friends or parents. Because the visual and psychological improvement following the operation is usually dramatic, otoplasty is rewarding to the patient, the family, and the surgeon (**Fig. 16.1**).

The predisposition to protruding ears tends to permeate a family's genetic tree, but with a varying degree of penetrance. In some cases an entire generation may be skipped. Some family members will have ears that look fairly normal, but others will have one or usually both ears that protrude, at least to some degree.

Even if only one ear appears to protrude excessively, it is usually necessary to correct both to obtain the desired surgical result.

For children to avoid classroom teasing and "nicknames," the surgery is preferably performed before they begin school. However, otoplasty can be performed at any age. By the age of 6, the ears have reached about 90% of their adult size. Little growth *of the ears* occurs after this time.

It is often helpful to teach patients and their families that, embryologically, the anterior one-half of the head develops from two opposing sides. In keeping with anatomical variations in other parts of the face and body, rarely are the two ears identical (prior to surgery). If they are not, chances are the ears will not be identical after surgery. It is crucial that patients and parents be advised of this fact. Let them know that—before birth, during embryonic development—ears exhibit none of the curves and creases seen at birth. Until the latter trimester of development, ears project straight out away from the head. Toward the end of gestation, however, the cartilages begin to curl, usually assume a position closer to the head, and develop the natural folds and convolutions. In patients whose ears unduly project from the head and lack the usual folds and convolutions, this aspect of the developmental process simply stopped short of completion.

The otoplasty procedure is designed to "complete" the developmental process by contouring the cartilage and positioning the ears closer to the head. Natural curvatures on the antihelix are generally created by placing sutures in the ear cartilages so that they can "heal" in their desired position over the ensuing weeks.

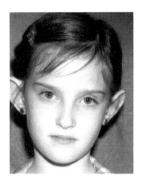 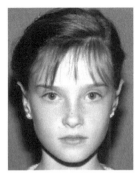

Fig. 16.1 **(a)** Large or protruding ears can be repositioned with the otoplasty procedure. **(b)** Although the size of the ears is not changed, they assume a much more natural relationship to the head.

Patients (parents in the case of minors) should also be advised that—when the ear cartilage is thick and strong—it tends to resist being repositioned and a "tuck" might be indicated in the future.

Patients are advised not to sleep on their ears and to avoid activities that could cause cartilage-contouring sutures to be stressed for at least 4 to 6 weeks.

A study performed in the 1980s by New York facial plastic surgeon Dr. Sidney Feuerstein demonstrated that after 6 weeks scar tissue—not sutures—held the ear in its new position. The takeaway message of Feuerstein's study is this: when performing otoplasty, use sutures that maintain tensile strength for 6 weeks, then dissolve. Permanent sutures are foreign bodies, subject to infection and extrusion.

17 Rejuvenizing the Aging Face: Facts and Myths

This chapter is designed to help facial surgeons address common questions and concerns posed by patients contemplating rejuvenation procedures. Specific procedures designed to accomplish rejuvenation are discussed in subsequent chapters 18–25.

To provide an algorithmic approach to facial rejuvenation surgery, I developed the following classification. It addresses the stages of aging and the surgical procedures that are available to stabilize or reverse them and should assist facial surgeons in providing "informed consent" to potential patients.

Facelift is the term commonly used to describe a surgical procedure better known in medical circles as "rhytidectomy" (the surgical removal/repositioning of loose, wrinkled skin of the face and neck). The procedure is designed to re-create the firmer, smoother face of youth. However, not all facelifts are the same—nor should they be! The reason is that *not all faces are the same.* And at different ages, the same face is a different face.

The *McCollough Facial Rejuvenation System* was introduced in 2012 in the peer-reviewed journal *Facial Plastic Surgery.*[1] The system comprises five general treatment plans:

- **Stage I (The Less Than 30 Facial Rejuvenation Plan)**: for the younger individual who has little or no loose skin and may require only liposuction to remove unwanted fat and bulges in the neck and lower cheeks.
- **Stage II (The 30-Plus Facial Rejuvenation Plan)**: for the patient who is beginning to notice sagging of the brows and cheeks, *but not the neck.* Whenever sagging tissues are present, facial muscles and fat must be repositioned into their more youthful relationships. In such cases a small amount of loose skin is removed.
- **Stage III (The 40-Something Facial Rejuvenation Plan)**: for the patient who exhibits sagging brows, cheeks, and neck. These patients may or may not need liposuction for contouring jowls and fullness under the chin. All, however, require suspension techniques to muscles and fat.
- **Stage IV (The 50-Something Facial Rejuvenation Plan)**: for the patient with *generalized* facial and neck sagging, with—or without—jowls and wrinkles

around the mouth. With more obvious muscle, fat, and skin laxity, more suspension of these structures is required.

- **Stage V (The 60-Plus Facial Rejuvenation Plan):** for the patient with *advanced* aging, coupled with sagging of all facial areas, including the forehead, brows, cheeks, and neck. At this stage in the aging process, deep folds develop in the groove between the nose and face, jowls droop below the jawline, and the muscles of the neck often produce stringlike bands that run vertically from the chin to the upper chest. Many of these patients are also beginning to exhibit wrinkles and blemishes over most of the face. Transcutaneous removal of skin and fat in the upper and lower eyelids is almost always indicated.[1]

■ Does Age Really Matter?

I rarely pay attention to a patient's chronological age. The reason is that individuals who share *the same chronological age* will exhibit more—or less—aging than their peers. Several factors contribute to this fact, including genetics, lifestyle, stress, nutrition, nicotine, and (excessive) alcohol use.

Surgery that addresses facial aging must focus on more than sagging skin of the cheeks and neck. For naturally enhanced faces, volume replacement and redistribution must be considered. While a facelift may play a significant role in a master plan, if the best results are to be obtained, more than traditional facelift surgery should be considered. Many patients benefit from work on the eyebrows and/or upper and lower eyelids to remove bags and sags in those regions. Those with wrinkles, acne scars, and sun-damaged skin should be advised that one of the level II or III skin resurfacing procedures mentioned in Chapters 21-24 could provide the "icing on the cake."

Some patients will require *liposuction* in the lower cheeks and neck. In fact, patients under the age of 40 might require *nothing more than* facial and neck liposuction, following which their youthful skin will "contract" to conform to the newly sculpted shape of the face and neck. And temporary injectable fillers can help bridge the gap until surgery can provide more permanent correction, or as "bridge alternatives" between "continuing maintenance" surgical procedures.

Depending on the length of time it takes a surgeon to perform individual elements of rejuvenating facial surgery, multiple procedures can be performed at the same time as the facelift, and without extending recovery times.

A good rule of thumb is to limit the total operating time to *less than 5 hours*, especially if surgery is being performed outside a hospital.

In the formative years of a facial surgeon's career, it is wise to exercise Ockham's logic: the simplest treatment plan is usually the correct one.

At *every stage* in a facial surgeon's career an irrefutable tenet of caring for patients applies: *diagnosis precedes treatment.* A corollary to this venerable principle is this: the *right* diagnosis, combined with the treatment(s) a surgeon is qualified to perform at a given career stage, on a particular face, is apt to yield happier outcomes. Based on these undeniable tenets, the only possible deduction is that a surgeon's ability to deliver optimal results on any given face improves with each passing year, with every face treated. Thus, in the formative years, "less is often better."

Not all faces should have *the same* treatment. Instead, a long-term rejuvenation plan should be considered *prior to* the initiation of treatment, even for treatments that promise only short-term benefits (i.e., injectables). Facial rejuvenation plans should be personalized and tailored to meet the needs and desires of each patient, at every stage of life. Each treatment plan must also coincide with the experience and skill of the surgeon.

Unfortunately, we live in a world with an appetite for instant gratification, even if it means *short-lived results.* That mind-set has found its way into the appearance-enhancement industry. The result is that commercialization (and not *condition-specific*, verifiable science) too often drives public demand. And in a rapidly changing society, demand tends to generate the opportunity for predatory exploitation.

In response to market-driven consumer demand, too many facial surgeons appear to be playing the role of *trend follower* rather than *leader.* For fear of losing patients to competing doctors, the tendency is to give patients *what they ask for*, rather than take the time to explain alternative methods of treatment and recommend *the best* alternative for each patient. The challenge is greater today because patients present with preconceived ideas and ask for therapeutic options television and print commercials prompt them to ask for.

Changes *within* the medical profession itself are also contributing to the dilemma. With the oncoming avalanche of regulated health care and declining imbursements from government and private health insurance companies, many doctors are turning to *cosmetic procedures* as a way to shore up consistently dwindling incomes.

Technology companies recognize the changes taking place throughout the health care industry. That industry appeals to doctors to include the products and machines they manufacture—laser treatments, injectable therapies, and "cookie cutter" types of surgical procedures, some of which can be "franchised." The imprudence in such a trend is rather obvious. Promoters prosper; physicians—and the patients they are entrusted to care for—pay the price.

Unfortunately, commercialized facelift procedures fall into the "one-size-fits-all" (or perhaps *fits none*) category. And some surgeons have been trained in only "one way" to perform the procedure, regardless of the conditions exhibited by the patients who entrust theirface to that practitioner. So facial rejuvenation is subject to the age-old truism that *if all one has is a hammer, everything takes on the shape of a nail.*

The fact is that aesthetic plastic surgery is very much an art form and can be tailored by an experienced surgeon/artist to meet the specific needs of each individual who presents for treatment.

The same face changes with advancing age. In one's late 30s the tissues of the brows, cheeks, and neck begin to descend from their youthful position, creating a "tired look." Alternating ridges and valleys create shadows in the face, and tissues begin to hang below the jawline and under the chin. With each passing year, these conditions progress, until the individual exhibits the undesirable characteristics of "old age." It is possible, however, *to prevent* these typical changes and to correct them as they occur. The "youth maintenance approach" addresses the signs of aging *as they occur* so that the individual never seems to age. The "rejuvenation approach" addresses the conditions of aging *after* they become obvious to the patient, and to others. Both approaches are effective. The bottom line is that surgery is available to either *retain* or *regain* a youthful and vibrant face.

■ When Is Facial Plastic Surgery Indicated?

The following questions are frequently asked—by patients and developing surgeons alike.

When is an often asked question. The best answer a facial surgeon can give is when sagging tissues of the face and neck or "bags" around the eyes are not temporary conditions relieved by rest, or when they become increasingly difficult to camouflage with cosmetics. When it comes to a specific age, the right answer is that one's *chronological age does not matter!*

As the life span lengthens in modern America, most people feel vigorous and energetic long after their appearance begins to deteriorate as a result of advancing years.

The onset of aging plays an important part in the personal and financial welfare of men and women from all walks of life. Almost everyone knows of people whose employment opportunities have been limited or curtailed because they "appear old," even though they might be more capable and competent than younger individuals.

For hundreds of years experts have confirmed that favors are granted to beautiful or handsome people. In Chapter 10 you were reminded that good looks affect school grades, enhance the probability of prosperity, determine who will be our friends, and shorten stays in mental hospitals.

The appearance of aging also imposes certain limitations in the area of social interests. Finally, the emotional impact of looking older than one feels can be disconcerting.

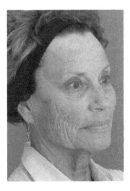
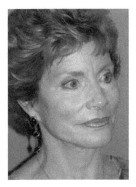

Fig. 17.1 **(a)** This woman had upper and lower blepharoplasty and lower and temporal, cheek, and neck facelift. **(b)** Several months later she had full face resurfacing with a combination chemical peel and dermabrasion to remove deep facial wrinkles.

There are two schools of thought: (1) to *preserve* one's youth and/or beauty by having problems corrected as they occur, or (2) to wait until the aging process has erased the appearance of both youth and beauty, then take measures to *recapture* that appearance with several surgical procedures. In short, choose between preventive maintenance and restorative rejuvenation (**Fig. 17.1**).

If a patient wishes to remain looking younger, the elite facial surgeon will explain that it is possible to perform a continuing series of relatively minor cosmetic surgery procedures as each of the irreversible changes of aging makes its appearance. With such a *maintenance program,* the patient can maintain a youthful appearance. Family, friends, and acquaintances are apt to remark that the patient doesn't seem to grow older. Today, most people choose this route. But in patients who didn't start such a preventive maintenance program when they were younger, a facial surgeon should outline a rejuvenation program to help the patients look as young and well as they feel.

■ Why All Faces Droop and Sag

In any given face, changes associated with aging do not occur all at once. Rather, they happen in a slowly progressive manner and involve all components of the face and body. There is no debate that human beings age differently. Patients frequently become aware of the changes over a 2- to 4-year period in their early 40s, occasionally sooner. They often tell me that it seemed as though things were aging well and then things seemed to change almost overnight, *especially following a period of intensive and prolonged stress.*

With aging, the skull becomes smaller, some fat is absorbed, and the skin loses much of its elasticity. As a result, the enveloping tissues, particularly in the face and neck, droop and sag. *The envelope becomes larger than its contents.* This phenomenon results in a series of events, including deepening of the lines of facial expression in the forehead and at the sides of the mouth; sagging of the eyebrows, which causes the eyes to appear smaller and crow's-feet to form at their corners; pouches or jowls forming along the jawline; and of course, development of the well-known "double chin."

At the same time, certain degenerative changes occur within the skin itself so that it seems to look "tired." In addition to the sagging, some faces become etched with wrinkles, especially those repetitively exposed to the sun and wind.

As occurs in other parts of the body, the muscles and tissues around the eyes eventually lose some of their tone so that a portion of the fat normally located inside the orbit around the eye bulges forward, or herniates, to produce the commonly seen "bags" or pouches. This condition can also be seen in younger people. "Circles" under the eyes may be a result of a shadow falling in the crease between mounds of pouches in the lower lid and cheek.

Finally, because of absorption of tissues in the upper lip and gums, the lips become thinner and the tip of the nose drops, causing it to appear larger and longer. Repositioning and supporting the tip of the nose can have dramatic and lasting effects on reversing this telltale sign of the aging process.

One needs only to study a child's face to see the physical characteristics that exemplify youth (fuller lips, larger eyes, arched eyebrows, smoother skin, and a shorter nose).

Each individual who wants to look "better" presents a different set of problems. This fact is why I created the "condition-specific" approach to facial rejuvenation. The corrective procedures indicated vary with each face, at every age. For example, one person may require only elevation of sagging eyebrows or improvement in the eyelids; a very young individual may need only correction of an early double chin with liposuction. On the other hand, a partial or complete face and neck lift followed in 3 to 6 months by a skin resurfacing procedure may be called for in more advanced cases.

When the skin is weather-beaten in appearance or has deep wrinkles, a chemical face peel, dermabrasion, and/or a laser resurfacing procedure may provide the icing on the cake (see Skin Rejuvenation, Chapter 20).

As a rule, a facelift, blepharoplasty, or submental lipectomy improves sags and bulges; resurfacing (laser, dermabrasion, and peeling) improves wrinkles and replaces sun-damaged skin (that is more prone to develop skin cancers) with more youthful and healthier skin.

■ Prevention or Rejuvenation?

There are two acceptable schools of thought. Some experts believe that as soon as aging signs appear, they should be corrected; thus patients will never appear as old as they are on the chronological scale. Most entertainment personalities or public figures have followed this principle. They have never allowed themselves *to look old.*

The alternative is to wait until the signs of aging are noticeable to have them corrected. Those who wait frequently regret not having had the surgery done earlier so that they could have enjoyed their more youthful look longer.

The motivation to look good is often rewarded in terms far beyond dollars. People who take pride in their health and pay attention to clothing, grooming, and overall personal appearance soon realize that exercise and proper nutrition can keep every part of the body other than the face toned up and looking more youthful than its chronological age. Regardless of what one might read or hear, *nothing short of surgery can help the face maintain that same youthful appearance.* Temporary "fixes" (neuromodulators and injectable fillers, facial exercises, electrical stimulation, acupuncture, creams, etc.) provide short-term improvement but will not correct the inevitable signs of aging.

■ Injectable Therapies

In Chapter 25, I provide a more detailed discussion on injectable therapies.

Temporary fillers dissolve within weeks to months, requiring multiple treatments, and may lead to problems. It took years for the medical profession to report on cases of skin necrosis following injectable fillers to the glabellar and nasal tip areas. The age-old adage "If it sounds too good to be true, it is usually is" applies to injectable treatments to treat the aging process. I feel that more predictable and time-tested procedures should be recommended to patients. *Quick fixes* generally lead to *quick returns* of the condition treated. Thus, the condition requires ongoing temporary treatments.

Many new tissue fillers are more promising than their predecessors. Neuromodulators (Botulinum Toxin type a) only treat conditions that occur with facial expression. They paralyze muscles and (for a while) prevent the wrinkles of expression from appearing. Concerns about atrophy of facial musculature following long-term, uninterrupted use of muscle-paralyzing agents linger.

Science-focused facial plastic surgeons are constantly investigating procedures, products, and techniques designed to provide the best result, with the least risks, with long-term benefits. My experience-based advice is to be slow to incorporate "new" products and technology into one's practice. In the long run, patients and colleagues alike appreciate—and reward—prudence in their appearance-enhancement providers.

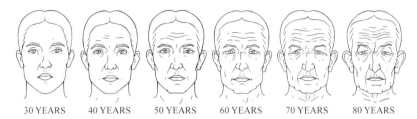

30 YEARS   40 YEARS   50 YEARS   60 YEARS   70 YEARS   80 YEARS

Fig. 17.2   This drawing demonstrates the changes that occur in the same face at 10-year intervals. Surgery can generally move one back one step, sometimes more, depending upon which procedures are performed.

■ Who Is a Candidate to Undergo Rejuvenation Procedures?

When is an often asked question. The answer is that when the face one sees in the mirror does not match the person one feels oneself to be, that is the time to consider facial plastic surgery.

Not everyone seeking an operation is an acceptable candidate. I usually advise against surgery in people with serious disease; those who are obese; those in whom preoperative laboratory tests or medical clearance (which I require) discloses conditions of concern; or prospective patients who have unrealistic expectations or inappropriate motivation. A prospective patient who cannot accept "less than perfection" as the goal and those who refuse to comply with my recommendations and the postoperative instructions I provide are also excluded.

■ What Can Surgery Do?

Patients must be told that cosmetic/aesthetic surgery turns back the clock; it does not stop the ticking. No operation or injectable product can prevent aging, but individuals who have undergone *surgery* to reverse the signs of aging that have occurred to that point in their life should never appear as old as they might have if the operation had not been done. Consider these two similar facts: Getting a haircut does not mean that another haircut will not become an option in the future. Trimming one's fingernails and toenails does not mean that the nails will not require attention as the days and weeks pass. The same principle applies to correcting the signs of aging that are present at the time a patient undergoes age management surgery. It is as though one's appearance is moved several years back on the "conveyor belt of time" (**Fig. 17.2**). However, the conveyor belt of aging continues to move *after* surgery.

The appropriate surgery might move patients back so that they could appear similar to the way they did years previously; in advanced cases patients can often look 10 to 15 years younger. I usually tell patients to pull out a photograph album and revisit photographs of themselves taken about 10 to 15 years previously. That is the appearance I will be attempting to achieve. They are generally relieved to know that I do not intend to give them the "plastic look" or the appearance of someone other than who they are. Their families are also relieved with such assurances.

■ Some Misconceptions

Much has been written in the lay press about aesthetic plastic surgery by non-physicians. In an attempt to write "something new" or to sensationalize the story, they have often written half-truths that have led to public misconceptions.

The following are some questions frequently asked by misinformed patients. The facial surgeon who can answer these questions with confidence and conviction will convert a higher percentage of consultations to surgery and lasting doctor-patient relationships.

Must I Have Another Facelift?

Many patients believe that once they have a facelift they *must* have another; otherwise they will look worse than if they had never had the first surgery. It is difficult to find the original source of this myth, but it is "out there." Facial surgeons who can tell patients that this has not been their experience will allay a lot of anxiety.

Patients can be told the following, however. It is true that a mini-lift (tuck-up) at a later date can improve *new* sagging that might occur with the normal aging process, but the patient's excessive skin *was removed* at the time of the original surgery and *that skin* is gone forever. The remaining tissues tend to age by the same natural process that led to the signs of aging corrected with the first facelift or eyelid lift (blepharoplasty).

I use the following scenario to assist in answering the question posed in the heading of this section: *After surgery*, the conveyer belt of time continues to move forward and the clock keeps ticking. At some point individuals will "catch up," once again, to their preoperative position. However, had surgery not been performed, they would have been farther down the line on the conveyor belt. Another helpful example is that when one trims one's nails, the nails do not remain at that length forever. They require maintenance to keep them at the desired length. And nails grow at different rates in different individuals. The best answer to "How long does a facelift last?" is *for the rest of the patient's life.* The patient *always* appears younger than had the patient not had surgery. This is not the case with temporary, injectable therapies.

I also find it helpful to explain that—during surgery—the excess skin and fatty tissues are *removed* and discarded. Those tissues that remain, however, continue to age naturally, and at a rate beyond the control of the facial surgeon.

An added point to emphasize here is that once breakdown of facial tissues begins, the aging process seems to accelerate—similarly to a snowball rolling downhill. The *rate of continuing aging* and sagging is dependent upon a variety of factors not under the control of the surgeon.

This is also a good time to remind patients that certain lifestyles and conditions tend to *speed up* the aging process: prolonged stress or illness in themselves or a loved one has always been known to hasten the signs of aging. I use the appearance of presidents when they are sworn into office and when they leave office. Most of them appear to be 10 to 12 years older after 4 years and 15 to 20 years older after 8 years. Patients clearly understand the comparison.

The teaching point message here is that whenever a facial surgeon can give real-life examples to which patients can relate to answer their questions, the answers sink in.

Will the Face Appear Stretched?

The unnatural, stretched, or "windblown" appearance frequently seen at the hands of some surgeons (and in some regions of the world) results from *how* the surgery was performed, not *that* the patient had a plastic surgery procedure. When patients demonstrate the "stretched look," the operating surgeon pulled the skin and underlying muscles *tightly* and *backward*. Another cause of a "stretched" face is *overvolumization* with injectables or fat grafting. My facelift techniques are specifically designed to avoid the "overoperated" or "plastic" look. I lift sagging tissues upward *and backward* at a vector of about 45°, thus placing the tissues back into hollowed areas where they rested several years previously. Directly vertical vectors and directly backward vectors are not recommended.

Facial surgeons can demonstrate (with the patient standing before a three-way mirror) how their procedures are designed to help safeguard against the justified concerns of telltale signs of plastic surgery for patients contemplating facelift and eyelid surgery.

What Should My Weight Be?

I prefer that my patients be well nourished prior to surgery. Crash diets tend to deplete the body of essential nutrients needed for proper healing and are not recommended. If the surgeon suspects that the patient is not in positive nitrogen balance or has a vitamin or mineral deficiency, it is possible to perform laboratory testing to identify such deficiencies.

In medical terms, weight loss occurs when the body goes into a *cannibalistic state* (negative nitrogen balance.) To heal properly from a surgical procedure the body needs to be in an *anabolic* state (positive nitrogen balance). Though I do not perform body plastic surgery, I have long had plastic surgeons in my clinics who do. It is well known among the circles of body plastic surgeons that patients who have achieved massive weight loss tend to heal poorly following procedures to remove the hanging skin that remains behind. Ockham's logic would suggest that it is because some of those patients never reset their metabolism from a cannibalistic state to an anabolic state.

The final teaching point of this section is this: I suggest to patients who lose weight prior to surgery to make sure they gain a pound or two back prior to surgery. That is a *clinical indication* that they have reset their metabolism. I also place all patients on pharmaceutical-grade nutritional supplements during the healing process.

Will Surgery Correct Laugh and Frown Lines?

Patients should know that neither surgery nor skin resurfacing can correct wrinkles that occur *only* during facial expressions. That's where neuromodulators enter the comprehensive treatment plan.

Creases around the eyes produced with smiling, forehead creases that occur with frowning, and vertical lines in the upper lip that occur with puckering the lips are due to the contraction of the muscles of facial expression. None of the *surgical* procedures discussed in this book are designed to eliminate these conditions. If wrinkles and creases are present *at rest,* then resurfacing the skin with chemical peeling, laser therapy, and/or dermabrasion may improve rhytids present *in the resting state.*

Can I Ever Get in the Sun Again?

Patients are often misinformed about the long-term restriction of activities following a skin resurfacing procedure. They have heard that once they have had a peel, dermabrasion, or a laser procedure, they can *never* get in the sun again, This has not been my experience.

While it is important that patients avoid sun exposure and use sunscreen products to protect their new "babylike" skin, they should avoid all potential skin irritants until *all pink discoloration* that occurs during healing has subsided. Patients should know that as long as the skin is pink, it is not totally healed. Logical sun exposure after the pink discoloration has subsided is allowed. It simply takes time for the new skin created by a resurfacing procedure to heal, longer to toughen or build up a natural resistance to sun and wind. The bottom line is that as long as the skin remains pink after a skin resurfacing procedure, it is subject to irritations and blistering.

Patients who have undergone skin resurfacing (laser, peeling, or dermabrasion) and who live (or recover) in the coastal areas are subject to the salty winds coming off the oceans or gulf. This, combined with additional sun exposure makes this group of patients more subject to prolonged redness and irritation after treatment. Absolute compliance with posttreatment instructions is the best way to ensure rapid healing and happier outcomes. If resurfacing procedures have not been performed, patients may be out of doors within a few days.

Skin care experts can also assist patients with a skin maintenance program designed to protect and preserve the more youthful skin achieved through resurfacing.

When Will I Be Presentable?

This is another common question asked by patients contemplating facial plastic surgery. Tell them that some degree of swelling follows any surgical procedure, that swelling and tightness are due to the new tissue fluids brought into the area by the body to promote healing, that increased blood supply to the region (required for healing) is responsible for the pink color of the skin and for some of the reddish "discoloration" associated with surgery, that bruising is the deposition of blood that oozes from blood vessels under the skin during surgery and afterward, and that when these "healing fluids" are no longer required, the tissues release the fluids and they are absorbed through the bloodstream. You can also tell them that blood vessels that dilate during the healing process to bring nutrients to the area through the bloodstream generally shrink when healing is complete. The exception is some venous vessels. Intense pulsed light therapy or conservative electrical hyfrecation can often resolve these issues.

Patients must be willing to accept temporary swelling, tightness, discoloration, and numbness that occur following such operations. Tell patients that, though these are usually disconcerting, most people feel the inconvenience is a negligible price to pay for the physical and psychological improvement they experience when healing is complete. Tell them that how quickly they heal depends, in part, on how carefully—and vigilantly—they follow "doctor's orders."

This is another opportunity to use an example to which patients can relate. I tell them that my pre- and postoperative routine is very much like a recipe. If a recipe is followed—to the letter—one generally knows what is going to come out of the oven. But if the recipe is altered, if the temperature setting is altered, or if the time the dish is left in the oven is altered, one does not know what may emerge from the oven. I tell them that their adherence to my instructions and admonitions will help determine how quickly—and well—they heal, and whether the results of their surgery will meet our mutual expectations.

Patients should also be told that when an incision is made through the full thickness of the skin, it can only heal by producing a scar, which mends the two edges together. Explain that every attempt is made (in the operating room and after) to keep the scars narrow and camouflaged in natural facial folds and creases or hidden by hairlines, but that lack of wound care and stressing an incision site after surgery will result in more visible scars. Tell patients that it is their job to help the surgeon help incisional scars to heal as well as possible.

Except in areas where antitension taping (with Steri-Strips™ [3M Corporate Center, St. Paul, MN] or paper tape) is prohibitive, I utilize this known method of helping scars heal. Incision sites are covered with antitension paper taping for a week. Tapes are removed for suture removal at a week, and the wound is retaped in an antitension manner for another week. Patients are instructed to apply antitension taping over the incision sites (where feasible) at bedtime for 6 weeks. Of course it is not feasible to tape incisions at the hairlines or around the ears or eyes as described above. Direct browlift and submental incisions (or any incision out of the face used to excise skin lesions or cysts or to revise an existing scar) to lend themselves to antitension taping as described above. From personal observations, I have been disappointed with over-the-counter scar prevention products. The "placebo effect" may be of some benefit. At least the patient gets the sense that "something" is being done to assist healing.

Patients should also be told that—during the initial healing period—all scars will be pink and somewhat swollen and lumpy, but that scars usually become less conspicuous with time, as they "mature." And ironically, scars mature faster in older people than in younger ones.

In most cases scars on the face and eyelids eventually become barely visible to the casual observer. At any rate, properly applied cosmetics and hairstyling after the operation can help camouflage them. If, during the healing process, it appears that a scar is thickening and it itches, dilute (5–10 mg/mL) intralesional injections of steroids and/or 5-fluorouracil (5-FU) may be helpful, at 3-week intervals.

Whether with incisional procedures or with skin resurfacing, the much-feared scar called a "keloid" is extremely rare on the face. Certainly, some people are more prone to scarring than others.

During the initial consultation, I tell patients that—after surgery—most patients are able to resume the bulk of their preoperative routine within 1 to 2 weeks, depending on which procedures are done. (It would be approximately 3 to 4 weeks following a skin resurfacing procedure.) Some makeup and hairstyling may be required for camouflaging the early signs of healing. I also recommend that patients consult with a trained aesthetician/skin care expert regarding makeup and skin care management. A systematic posttreatment skin care program administered by a trained and experienced aesthetician can not only speed up the healing process in most cases, but also help maintain the desired appearance of healthier, happier skin for years to come.

■ Will I Be Happier after Surgery?

Most patients are happier when they appear younger and more rested; however, an operation alone is incapable of turning an unhappy person into a happy person. It's not that simple. One's attitude toward life and how one deals with one's own special set of circumstances is the key to happiness. I would also stress that the caring demeanor of and encouraging words from the facial surgeon and the surgeon's staff can help build self-esteem in patients who have undergone life-changing events.

In preoperative literature I provide for patients, I inform them that they should not expect plastic surgery to solve personal, domestic, or professional problems, nor should they seek universal approval from family, friends, or acquaintances before or after surgery.

The decision to have plastic surgery is a personal choice, based upon realistic expectations and mutual trust between the patient and the surgeon. In uncomplicated cases, patients are generally satisfied with their results and recommend surgery to friends and family.

The final result of any treatment depends upon a myriad of factors, risks, and imponderables. I tell patients that should they have questions after surgery, I urge them to contact me. I tell them that if they are displeased with the outcome, I want to be the first to know, so that we can work through the issue and make it better, if indicated. This makes for long-lasting doctor-patient relationships and is one of those "practice-building secrets" that facial surgeons do not usually learn, unless they serve a fellowship with a colleague who understands the "art" of creating—and maintaining—interpersonal relationships of a lasting nature.

■ Can Multiple Procedures Be Performed at the Same Time?

In my practice patients are informed that it is possible for them to have several procedures performed during the same operating room experience.

A patient's health, the types of procedures, and the schedules of the surgeons may determine *how much* can be done. In the preceding sentence, I say "surgeons" because I have—in my practice—a plastic surgeon who performs body procedures, and we often work at the same time. He often performs a body procedure at the same time I am performing a facial procedure.

■ References

1. McCollough EG, Ha CD. The McCollough Facial Rejuvenation System: expanding the scope of a condition-specific algorithm. Facial Plast Surg 2012;28(1):102–115

18 Blepharoplasty

Wrinkles, loose skin, and bulges occur as a result of hereditary factors and the aging process. Pouches or bags of the upper and lower lids are generally due to weakening of the tissues of the orbital septum and protrusions of intraorbital fat (**Fig. 18.1**). In some cases edema in the periorbital tissues contribute to the condition. In my practice, fat bulges are generally removed. When conservatism is exercised, I have not found an indication for fat repositioning (the sub–orbicularis oculi fat [SOOF]). A good rule to follow is to not remove fat that lies deep to the infraorbital rim. only that which protrudes beyond it.

Fatty pouches are sometimes seen in the 20- to 30-year age group, occasionally younger, and can often be corrected at that time. After addressing possible medical reasons for these bulges (allergies, kidney and thyroid disease), there is little rationale to wait for some arbitrary age before having surgery. When the problem exists, it should be corrected (Fig. 18.2).

Upper lid surgery is usually performed at the same time as the lower lid surgery, but either can be done as an isolated procedure. Upper and lower eyelid plastic surgery may also be performed with a facelift, browlift, or other surgery. When a skin–muscle technique is used in the lower lids, a level II chemical peel may be performed at the same time, as long as the peel solution does not extend to the incision site.

It is not the intent of this chapter, or others, to describe details of my surgical techniques. They are provided in other publications and video demonstrations. Rather, the purpose of this book is to discuss the art of practice development and management, skills not generally learned through traditional training methods.

In upper lid blepharoplasty a preoperative determination is made about the excess or overlapping skin that frequently obliterates the natural crease above the lashes. The excess skin and fat are removed, and the incision sites are closed with delicate sutures. Magnification often assists the surgeon in absolute approximation of the skin edges, for better postoperative scars.

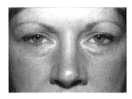
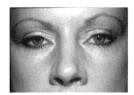

Fig. 18.1 Drooping, heavy tissues around the eyes can be removed with the upper and lower lid plastic surgery procedure blepharoplasty to remove the "tired look."

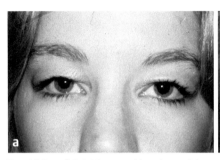
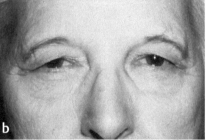

Fig. 18.2 **(a)** A 17-year-old patient with excessive upper lid skin. **(b)** A 70-plus-year-old patient with excessive skin of her upper lids and drooping brows.

■ Transconjunctival Blepharoplasty

In some patients the herniated fat producing "bags" or bulges in the lower lid can be removed *without making an incision in the skin.* The incision is made behind the lower lid, thereby eliminating a visible scar.

It is not possible to remove loose skin or sagging wrinkles when this method is used, unless an external incision is also made in the eyelid skin, usually at the level of the lower border of the tarsus. In most cases this anatomical landmark coincides with the first rhytid in the lower eyelid skin.

Skin resurfacing (laser, peeling, or dermabrasion) can also be performed at the same time as transconjunctival blepharoplasty to minimize many of the fine wrinkles. These options should be discussed with patients during the initial consultation. They should know that there is more than one way to address their concerns. It is perfectly acceptable, however, for a facial surgeon to offer a "recommended" course of treatment.

■ Transcutaneous Lower Lid Surgery

Lower eyelid blepharoplasty may also be performed by making an incision in the skin below the lower lashes (in my technique, in the first wrinkle, which—as stated above—also coincides with the inferior border of the lower eyelid tarsus). Making the incision at this level preserves the pretarsal orbicularis portion of the orbicularis oculi muscle, an integral component of the lower eyelid suspensory complex.

Additionally, the undisturbed skin bridge left between the incision and the lid margin has the ability to "stretch" (as does all skin placed on tension) in case aggressive removal of the skin inferior to the incision is performed or unanticipated scarring should develop in the subdermal plane during the healing process. Preservation of the pretarsal orbicularis also tends to provide a more natural-appearing lower eyelid.

In my experience, the combination of the afore-referenced precautionary measures makes it unnecessary to perform suspensory techniques, unless the patient is found—preoperatively—to have an atonic lower lid sling or hammock.

Access to bulging fat can be readily accomplished by a "skin–muscle" elevation, in which the orbicularis oculi muscle inferior to the incision can be lifted in conjunction with the skin. Or the fat can be accessed by elevating skin only and dividing the orbicularis muscle with blunt dissection, just superior to the infraorbital rim of the orbital skeleton.

I recommend and practice conservative fat removal. Only fat that protrudes *outside* the orbital rim is removed. Meticulous cauterization of the remaining stalk with bipolar cautery is recommended. I neither recommend, nor practice, venturing into the orbit to remove fat. In my experience it is not *that* fat was removed, but that *excessive amounts* of fat were removed, that results in a "hollow eye" postoperative appearance and deepening of the so-called tear trough.

Once bulging fat is removed, the skin (or skin–muscle) flap is gently placed back in position. Only overlapping portions of skin or muscle are conservatively trimmed. Small delicate sutures are used to close the lower lid incisions. Once again, magnification results in more accurate approximation.

Because the skin at the outer corners of the eye is thicker than in other parts of the lid, it takes a little longer for the incisional scar in that area to soften and flatten after surgery. Sometimes, intralesional "droplet" injections of dilute cortisone (triamcinolone 5.0–7.5 mg/mL) speed the healing process along. As in all areas, caution should be exercised. Overly aggressive injection of steroids can dissolve tissues in the subcutaneous plane and result in dimpling.

With the passage of time, the incision lines of the upper and lower lids are difficult—if not impossible—to see with the naked eye.

As a rule, eyelid procedures are associated with minor disability and allow one to return to routine living after a few days using cosmetics and sunglasses.

Most patients tell me that there is no pain in the operated areas during the postoperative period. Each operation is followed by varying degrees of swelling and/or discoloration, most of which usually subsides within 7 to 10 days. By this time, too, the scars can be camouflaged by makeup.

When wrinkling of the lower lid and lateral orbital region is pronounced, I frequently recommend skin resurfacing to cause further tightening of the skin and improvement of fine wrinkles or crow's-feet, but not over a *skin-only* flap elevation, unless the surgeon has years of experience in chemical skin resurfacing. A level II Baker's peel may be performed with transconjuctival and skin–muscle blepharoplasty. However, due to the fact that some skin tightening occurs with these peels, it is recommended that the amount of skin excised should be taken into account.

The healing period for this level of skin resurfacing, however, is 2 to 3 weeks (as it is with any level II peeling procedure). Some pink can persist for up to 8 weeks—longer if the patient fails to comply with postoperative instructions and precautions.

Insurance does not ordinarily cover surgical fees and hospitalization expenses for cosmetic surgery. However, in patients who have *extreme* amounts of overhanging tissues producing "hooding," I request a consultation from an eye specialist. If the (visual fields) examination demonstrates visual impairment, a portion of the fees for "functional" upper lid surgery may be covered by medical insurance. In my experience, it is becoming more and more difficult to convince insurance companies to cover costs for functional eyelid surgery. When insurance companies agree to participate, reimbursement fees are a fraction of charges.

I have yet to encounter a case where excess skin and fat in the *lower lid* impaired a patient's vision; however, if I need to do a procedure to support/suspend a lax or drooping lower lid that contributes to "dry eyes," insurance may defray some of the costs for this portion of the lower lid operation.

Patients are advised to divulge any history of eye disease or history of visual problems so that they may be evaluated prior to surgery. Documentation of a patient's ability to read *with each eye* should be recorded prior to surgery, even if it is to read a printed form prepared by the surgeon's staff.

I recommend patients have an eye examination prior to eyelid surgery. I ask them to have their eye doctor send a report of the findings to me. I also offer to assist them in obtaining an appointment if they should have a problem obtaining one right away.

At times the curtain of skin hanging from the upper eyelid may be partially due to sagging *of the eyebrows*. In such cases, it may be necessary to advise elevation and support to the brows and forehead at the same time the upper lid plastic surgery is performed (see Chapter 19).

◼ The Other "Bulge"

Blepharoplasty is designed to correct conditions found *within* the anatomical confines of the bony rims of the eye socket.

Patients often ask if lower lid surgery removes or improves the swollen, puffy areas that sometimes develop beneath the lower lid and over the cheek (malar) bones. The generic answer is *no*. These bulges are thought to be caused by uncontrolled fluid accumulation in the tissues. They are, in essence, "a reservoir of edema." In some cases the edema is a result of allergies, chronic sinus disease, or fluid retention from excessive salt or yeast intake. Patients should be advised to notice and document days when the edema is most pronounced and reflect on food/drink intake and activities.

Direct excision may remove these unwanted edematous tissues, but is not indicated unless they become quite large festoons. The resultant scar may be imperceptible, but sometimes requires dermabrasion at a later time. Patients upon whom I have performed this procedure are much happier with thread-thin scars than the bags they were unable to camouflage.

19 The Eyebrow Lift

Drooping of the eyebrows is frequently one of the first signs of aging. This condition is often overlooked because most patients are unaware of the problem and the degree of improvement its correction can provide (**Fig. 19.1**).

A heavy eyebrow causes the upper lids to drop or descend until, in the advanced stages, eyelid skin can touch or overlap the eyelashes.

Patients often complain that their eyes appear to be getting smaller or deeper set and that (in women) eye makeup usually ends up high on the upper part of the lids within a short while after it has been applied. Drooping eyebrows definitely contribute to the dreaded "tired look."

In some cases, a patient's subconscious need to contract muscles in the forehead to lift a drooping brow can contribute to headaches. I explain this phenomenon in the following manner: Any muscle that is contracted over a protracted period of time fatigues. Fatigued muscles often cramp. And a cramp in the area of the forehead is called a "headache." Surgical eyebrow lifting can alleviate or reduce (on a long-term basis) the incidence of headache precipitated by a drooping eyebrow. Neuromodulators can do so on a temporary basis. And, on the subject of headaches, Chapter 12 (Nasal Plastic Surgery: Rhinoplasty) addresses an often unrecognized and correctable cause of headaches—impaction of the nasal septum against a turbinate.

Browlift surgery may be incorporated into forehead lifting. *In men*, I usually prefer direct excision of a measured section of skin above the drooping section of the brow. The excision lines used to remove forehead skin are placed *on either side of* (but not within) the most prominent rhytids in the forehead and beveled so that closure everts the skin edges (**Fig. 19.2**)

Following surgery, the wound is cross-taped in an antitension manner for a week. Sutures are removed at that time and the wound is retaped for another week. Patients are instructed on how to apply antitension taping each evening before going to bed and anytime they are "around the house" for the day. If antitension taping is appropriately applied for 4 to 6 weeks, the scars are generally imperceptible. In fact, they are usually less noticeable than the rhytids that were incorporated within the section of skin removed.

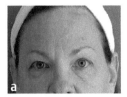
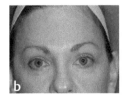

Fig. 19.1 **(a)** Heavy or low-set brows can give one a "tired" or "stern" look, **(b)** but a browlift can restore them to their proper position, resulting in a more alert and youthful appearance. The incisions in this direct browlift are immediately above the brow hairs but are easily camouflaged.

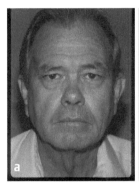
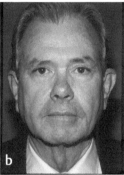

Fig. 19.2   (a) Prior to a browlift. (b) After the browlift.

Supraperiosteal undermining of the skin *inferior to the excision* is performed to the supraorbital rim. Doing so frees the arcus. Then subperiosteal undermining is carried forward into the upper eyelid for approximately 1 cm. The brow is advanced superiorly and the wound closed in three layers, taking great care to evert the skin edges.

Direct (midforehead) lifting and pre- and posthairline procedures "lift" the brow, upper lid, and surrounding tissues. Each technique usually results in eyes that appear larger, more rested, and more youthful. It should be emphasized that overcorrection of the brows in a male patient will have a tendency to "feminize" the periorbital region. In men, the brow should be positioned to lie at the level of the supraorbital rim. In a woman, however, the ability to visualize the supraorbital rim beneath the brow gives an aesthetically pleasing appearance.

Following eyebrow surgery, there is often lessening of the deeper crow's-feet found next to the *lateral corners* of the eye. However, for the best result, crow's-feet seen "at rest" may require a skin resurfacing procedure. Neuromodulators can be used to minimize rhytids that ordinarily occur with facial expression.

An eyebrow lift will not correct either excess skin or pouching caused by fat herniation at the inner corners of the upper lids, and it will not have any appreciable effect on lower lid conditions. On the other hand it can be, and often is, effectively combined with surgery designed to improve problems in those regions.

In female patients, I ordinarily prefer to accomplish the eyebrow lift in conjunction with the temporal or forehead portion of the facelift, but in some cases it may be performed as an independent procedure.

Smaller incisions with (and without) the use of an endoscope—and coupled with interruption of some of the muscles that create deep creases and wrinkles—can be used in some cases. The downside of any *post*hairline incisional technique is that the hairline is raised, at least, to the same degree that the brows are lifted—sometimes more.

For rejuvenating the forehead and glabellar areas, I prefer the trichophytic forehead lift. When it is performed properly, hair will grow through (and below) the scar, thereby making the scar a nonissue.

When deep glabellar creases are present, the corrugator muscles may be excised. In recent years, it has become recommended not to inject "fillers" into glabellar creases. Cases of skin necrosis have been documented. I prefer placement of a small strip of fascia in a pocket made through a small stab wound at the inferior end of the crease. Some 17 years of experience in doing so has proven rewarding to surgeon and patient alike.

Within and at the edges of hairlines closure is accomplished with stainless steel staples, between which a running 5–0 "fast-absorbing" plain catgut suture is used for more optimal apposition at the hairline.

20 The Facelift Operation

■ Rhytidectomy

The Greek word for wrinkle is *rhytid* and the suffix *ectomy* means "to remove or extract"; thus the term *rhytidectomy.* The layperson's name for rhytidectomy is "facelift."

The term *facelift* is often inappropriately used to reference *total facial rejuvenation,* which—in reality—consists of eyelid surgery, facelift, and perhaps skin resurfacing. Facial surgeons know these facts, but it is often helpful to explain them to patients during the initial consultation or with printed materials.

Patients should also be informed that a facelift comprises four parts: forehead, temporal, cheek, and neck lifts. Each of these components can stand alone or be performed in conjunction with another. The exception—in my practice—is that, at least, a partial lower cheek lift is usually required to correct bunching of neck skin advanced into the region just anterior to the lobule of the ear during a neck lift.

While a facelift provides the necessary foundation for rejuvenation of the face and neck, other procedures add the "finishing touches."

The goal of each component of the facelift operation is to reposition and remove the signs of aging caused by sagging of loose skin, muscles, and fatty tissues.

Facelift surgery *does not correct* aging lower eyelids. In fact, after a well-performed cheek lift, excessive skin of the lower lid is often more pronounced so that lower eyelid blepharoplasty, skin resurfacing, or both may be required. This is the best argument for performing blepharoplasty *after* the facelift part of a combined facial rejuvenation procedure. In the upper eyelid, less skin removal is necessary after a well-performed forehead/temporal browlift.

Although there is not uniform agreement on the specific techniques employed by facial surgeons, the facelift operation has become one of the most popular cosmetic operations performed in the head and neck. The reason is that as medical advances and new technology increase the average life span, many women, *and men*, find that they look older than they feel, physically and mentally. The social stigma previously associated with having plastic surgery is no longer a deterrent. However, when the surgery is performed in such a manner that patients demonstrate the signs of "overly done" surgery, friends and acquaintances are less apt to seek plastic surgery and the entire specialty of facial surgery is affected in a negative manner.

Still, men and women from all walks of life are seeking ways to look as good as they feel. It behooves all facial plastic surgeons to teach and perform techniques that give "natural" and "unoperated" results. The techniques I use, develop, and advocate are designed and dedicated to that end.

Facelifts may be done for one of two reasons. The first is to help *prevent* the advancement of aging, that is, to help relatively young individuals (around the age of 40) to maintain a youthful appearance. The second reason is to help patients with advanced signs of aging appear younger, fresher, and more rested—in short, to help one recapture the appearance enjoyed 10 to 15 years previously.

Naturally, everyone contemplating a facelift is interested in how much improvement they can expect, and for what duration. The amount of improvement depends on the condition of the skin and the degree of wrinkling and sagging present; if the visible signs of aging are excessive, the results may be dramatic—approaching the 15-year goal. If sagging is occurring prematurely and the operation is being done to attempt to *keep* the patient looking young, the improvement may be more subtle. People may remark that the face "looks more alive, rested, and fresher." Some people look as though they have lost weight because the heaviness along the jawline and in the neck is improved.

■ How Long Does a Facelift Last?

The following are some of the comments I use to answer questions asked by prospective patients.

The fact is that a facelift lasts *for a lifetime*, in that patients will always appear younger than had they not undergone the procedure. The duration of the results noticed within the first year after surgery cannot always be accurately predicted. Results will vary depending upon the specific surgical maneuvers taken by the surgeon, for example, whether liposuction was performed to remove portions of unwanted fat, whether superficial musculoaponeurotic system (SMAS) imbrication was performed and the manner in which the SMAS was suspended, and whether incisions were extended to adequately remove redundant skin.

If, preoperatively, wrinkling or sagging is severe, years will pass before the condition again becomes *as advanced* as before surgery. If the natural degenerative process in the skin is occurring rapidly due to poor health or stress, wrinkling and sagging will also accumulate more rapidly. This is precisely when "tuck-up" or "maintenance" procedures are helpful.

Liposuction can permanently remove unwanted fat cells from the neck and jawline. That it can means that the surgeon must be aware of regions of the face, neck, and subdermis that require fat to provide aesthetically pleasing volume and avoid overly aggressive removal. A thin layer of fat is necessary between the dermis and underlying musculature. Removal of buccal fat (a technique advocated in some circles in the past) is not recommended. In later years, this pad of fat is needed to avoid extreme hollowing of the midface.

When combined with tightening sagging muscles and skin in patients undergoing facial plastic surgery, liposuction can improve the results along the jawline and submental region by as much as 20 to 25%. When good skin tone is present and very little drooping is noted, the lower one-half of a face that is simply "fat" may be improved with liposuction alone.

In ideal cases, however, a more youthful appearance following a facelift can be enjoyed for 5 to 10 years. No operation can permanently *prevent* aging, but patients should *never* appear as old as they might have if the operation had not been done.

When proper attention is paid to the SMAS, sagging tissues in the brows, face, and neck noticed *after* a facelift are a result of the continuation of the aging process. When sagging becomes a problem again, a tuck-up procedure can be done that may provide dramatic and long-lasting improvement. I have patients for whom I have relied on "tuck" procedures to help them maintain a more youthful look for nearly 4 decades. Some would consent to surgery every year or so, if I would agree to perform it when they asked for it. It is my practice to delay additional procedures until I feel they are warranted. Because I established the doctor-patient relationship discussed in this book very early in the process, patients will concede to my recommendations.

For the best results, every patient should be evaluated within a year or two following surgery. A tuck-up may or may not be considered at this time. Aggressive lifting of facial tissues results in a "stretched" or "windblown" appearance, a condition that can—and should—be avoided.

The foundation created by the initial facelift creates the desired situation for a tuck-up. The thin layer of scar that is formed in the subcutaneous layer at the time of initial undermining and lifting provides additional strength when suspending the deeper tissues of the face during maintenance surgery.

Patients should know that it is not *necessary*, however, to have additional cosmetic surgery. The tuck-up is simply part of an elective alternative in a comprehensive "maintenance program."

In a Nutshell

In general, a facelift helps turn back the clock by about 10 years in most patients (**Fig. 20.1**). It does not *stop* the ticking. Excess skin and fat in the neck and lower jaw is removed at surgery. Any slack seen in the postoperative period is a result of *continued* aging and breaking down of the skin that remains. Had the surgery not been performed, the patient would have developed the "new" sags on top of the "old" sags that were removed at surgery. Tuck-ups help maintain a youthful appearance in the patient who *chooses* to have additional surgery. Tuck-ups are generally less extensive, less expensive, and quite effective.

■ Who Should Undergo a Facelift?

Men and women from all walks of life are opting to have facelifts; however, not everyone seeking rehabilitation of the aging skin of the face and neck is an acceptable candidate for surgery. Those with known serious medical problems are usually excluded. Patients who are obese or who have a short, thick neck have little chance for a worthwhile result. Those who are using—and have a long-standing history of using—nicotine products tend to heal poorly.

The severe "turkey gobbler" deformity that occurs in the neck of some individuals may best be corrected by a *direct excision* of the skin using a submental midline incision with a single small "**Z**-plasty" placed at the cervicomental angle. This procedure is generally reserved for male patients who resist conventional facelift and neck lift procedures.

■ Skin Rejuvenation

Smoother, wrinkle-free skin is a goal sought by patients and doctors alike. However, the cosmetic industry of the 21st century offers a plethora of

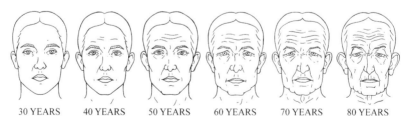

30 YEARS   40 YEARS   50 YEARS   60 YEARS   70 YEARS   80 YEARS

Fig. 20.1   The aging process (life's conveyor belt of time). This drawing demonstrates the changes that occur in the same face at 10-year intervals. Surgery can generally move one back one step, sometimes more, depending upon which procedures are performed.

products and procedures that, unfortunately, promote unrealistic expectations. A good rule for facial surgeons is to remind prospective patients that "superficial" treatments tend to *polish* the skin (leaving behind all the underlying conditions of aging), while deeper-penetrating treatments (that take at least 2 weeks to heal) actually *create new collagen and elastic tissues below the surface.*

To help clear up some of the confusion about skin rejuvenation procedures, I have developed a classification that accurately describes the extent to which facial skin should be—and can be—exfoliated. It is important to emphasize to patients that the end result of a skin exfoliating product or resurfacing procedure is directly proportional to *the depth (or penetration) of treatment,* meaning that deeper-penetrating treatments (although they require longer healing times) tend to yield better and longer-lasting results.

The microscopically *thin*, outermost layer of skin (epidermis) can clearly be removed with exfoliating cosmetics that contain diluted retinoic acid or glycolic, salicylic, or some related acid. These products tend to "polish" the skin, much in the same manner as furniture polish makes furniture shine, for a short while.

Another method of removing superficial layers of skin is with lasers, *micro*dermabrasion, or stronger concentrations of the acid preparations mentioned above. These procedures are often provided in spa settings. Daily use of a Buf-Puf sponge (3M Consumer Healthcare Division, St. Paul, MN) or exfoliating brush can provide many of the same results as *micro*dermabrasion.

The crucial point to remember is that *none of the aforementioned level I treatments penetrate into the deeper (or dermal) layers.* Because they do not, they are unable to reverse severe sun damage, blemishes, or wrinkles. *To have any long-lasting effect on these unwanted conditions, the treatment must extend into the upper level of dermis.* And even if treatment does extend to the dermal layer, it is important to keep in mind that *the methods* of removing or exfoliating skin are (more often than not) overexaggerated and overcommercialized. The truth is that the end result depends on *in whose hands any given technology is placed.*

Whether the doctor uses lasers, dermabrasion, chemical peeling, or a combination of all three, it is the *depth* or *penetration* to which the doctor carries the treatment (and not *the type of technology the doctor uses)* that determines the success (or failure) of any skin rejuvenation procedure. And keep in mind that "fractionated" resurfacing technology means that only fractions of the area are treated. Predetermined *non*treated parts of the same area are factored into the technology. The explanation for shorter "downtime" is that only half of the treatment load is delivered.

When considering a resurfacing procedure on any patient, the first step is to conduct a scientific skin analysis. Doing so determines the current stage of the skin *within each region of the face.* On *the same* face, skin thickness, solar damage, acne scarring, or wrinkling may differ; therefore, the treatment required for each area should be adjusted to the conditions that exist in each facial region. Said another way, the first—and often the most crucial—step in maintaining or enhancing the appearance of a patient's skin is to determine which areas require treatment and which areas should be left undisturbed, at least for the time being. For example, a patient may choose to treat the lines around the upper and lower lip, or wrinkles around the eyes, and leave other areas of the face alone. In other cases, it may be best to resurface the entire face. When you do this, the newly resurfaced skin blends into the various facial aesthetic units. An experienced facial surgeon can demonstrate the various aesthetic units (regions) of each patient's face in a mirror and recommend the most appropriate treatment modality for each.

III Minimally Invasive and Noninvasive Therapies

21 Advanced Skin Rejuvenation

The procedures described on the following pages have been called "nonsurgical facelifts." They are described in much greater detail in a textbook coauthored by me and Dr. Phillip R. Langsdon.[1]

I developed the following skin rejuvenation classification system:

- **Level I:** These treatments are often offered by nonsurgeons, frequently in a spa setting. Patients are able to return home or to work or play immediately. Little or no healing time is required. Level I treatments tend to "polish" the skin for a few weeks, but have essentially no long-term benefits. The exception to the above rule is that some topical products (e.g., hydroquinone) can improve dyschromic areas; however, the practitioner should consult the medical literature for recommended concentrations, combinations, and length of use.
- **Level II:** These skin resurfacing procedures are generally offered by facial surgeons and dermatologists. More layers of damaged and wrinkled skin are removed with these deeper (dermis-level) treatments. Healing generally requires about a week. Level II procedures are generally recommended for patients less than 50 years old or those with minimal to moderate sun damage and wrinkling.
- **Level III:** These procedures should be performed by experienced facial surgeons or surgically oriented dermatologists. Level III resurfacing procedures are the most effective methods of removing *severely* sun damaged, blotchy skin and deeper wrinkles. Healing time is longer—generally 2 to 3 weeks. However, results are long lasting and often dramatic. Although in most full-face resurfacing procedures I rely on a combination of chemical peeling and dermabrasion, long-term skin tightening along the jawlines is obtained when the cheek regions are treated with Baker's formula peel solution.

Different parts of the same face generally require differing levels or depths of treatment. For example, the thin skin of the eyelids may not tolerate the same level of treatment that the thicker skin of the forehead, nose, lips, and chin may require. An experienced surgeon will know how to vary the depth of the treatment to meet the specific needs of each patient.

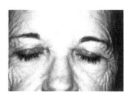 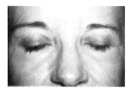

Fig. 21.1 (a) Prior to chemical peeling and brow lift. **(b)** After chemical peeling and brow lift.

While varying degrees of skin tightening occur with deeper (level II and III) resurfacing procedures, it is my opinion that the term *facelift* should be reserved for the procedures described in Chapter 20.

Creative formulas and methods of applying exfoliating solutions do not change the fact that the ingredients cause a separation of the upper layer of skin, which "peels" or "sheds" within a few days.

Varying layers of skin are removed by chemical peeling, dermabrasion, and laser resurfacing. Each seems to have unique qualities and benefits. An experienced surgeon must be able to explain to the patient which procedures might be the most advantageous in the patient's unique set of conditions, and in that surgeon's hands.

With all skin resurfacing methods, layers of the sun-damaged, wrinkled, or scarred skin are removed. However, only with deeper (level II and III) procedures are *new* collagen and elastic fibers produced in the deeper layers of skin. As a result, some tightening of facial tissues occurs, but not to the extent that can be accomplished with surgical removal through conventional facelift and eyelid lift techniques (**Fig. 21.1, Fig. 21.2**).

Superficial (level I) peels do *not* produce long-term improvement in the quality and texture of the skin and should be viewed as "polishing or pigmentation-lightening agents." As with any polishing agent, the results are not permanent and must be repeated every several weeks. Level I resurfacing procedures are often helpful as *adjuncts* to the level II and III methods herein described, but *only after healing is complete*—said another way, when *all pink coloration* from a *healing* level II or level III peel subsides. Most spas offer level I peels, unless a qualified—and properly licensed—medical professional is involved.

■ Treatment for Wrinkles

Neither a facelift, nor eyelid surgery (blepharoplasty), nor a browlift will eliminate wrinkles of weather-beaten skin, the horizontal creases of the forehead, crow's-feet that occur around the eyes, or the vertical wrinkles of the upper and lower lips. *Keep in mind that surgery is designed to improve sags and bulges, while level II and III resurfacing improves wrinkles.*

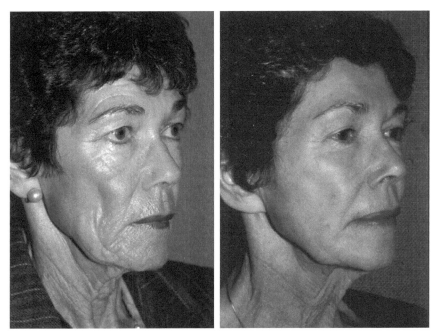

Fig. 21.2 (a) Prior to full face chemical peel. **(b)** After full face chemical peel. No other procedure was performed.

Combination treatment programs are often recommended. For example, a level II or III chemical peel or laser exfoliation might be performed for peri*oral* rhytids, a level II chemical peel for peri*orbital* rhytids, and dermabrasion for cheek skin scarred from acne or nasal skin exhibiting varying degrees of rhinophyma.

Level II and III resurfacing may improve the diffuse patchy pigmentation of the facial skin that sometimes accompanies and follows pregnancy or contact dermatitis. They may also help the "dark circles" that some people have under their eyes, but only *if the circles are caused by skin containing patchy areas of excessive melanin.*

Skin resurfacing may be done only in specific regions of the face (e.g., around the lips, around the eyes). It can be an indispensable adjunct to facelift and eyelid plastic surgery in an overall facial rejuvenation program. Until a facial surgeon has performed hundreds of level II or III skin resurfacing procedures, it is advisable to *wait 3 to 6 months before resurfacing areas in which skin is tightened with surgery.*

Some skin types are more favorable for treatment than others; fair complexions tend to respond better than dark ones. Thick, tough, more *deeply etched, or oily skins may require a two-staged approach for the best results* (e.g., a second resurfacing procedure or touch up of several areas at a later time). As with painting a roughly textured wall, deep creases and scars may require a touch-up.

Resurfacing alone is not indicated as the treatment of choice for sagging tissues. Although the new skin has better elasticity, stage IV and V facial aging requires surgery (see Chapter 20). Even so, after resurfacing, I have seen *additional tightening* in the skin in patients who underwent prior facelift surgery.

Skin resurfacing is considered a surgical procedure; therefore, the risks that apply to surgery must be considered and discussed. For full-face resurfacing, I utilize the same operating room facilities and anesthesia protocols employed for other facial surgical procedures.

Patients are warned that taking female hormones or birth control pills for approximately 6 months after a resurfacing may lead to hyperchromatic changes in skin pigmentation or color. Patients who feel they must take hormones usually do so without incurring any problems. Skin bleaching preparations that contain retinoic acid and hydroquinone can often be helpful in reducing posttreatment pigmentation, should it occur.

Vigilance in postoperative care cannot be overemphasized. In my practice, I give patients both printed and oral instructions to assist them in caring for their new, delicate skin and have them return frequently during the first week or so. When return visits are not possible, they e-mail photographs on a daily basis so that I can monitor their healing.

During the healing process, the patient's skin will be much like that of a baby. It takes time for the new skin to toughen and tolerate direct sun, wind exposure, and many skin care products. Because it is "new" skin, the texture and color will be somewhat different from that which has not been resurfaced. Makeup can generally be worn after 3 weeks and will camouflage any remaining color contrasts.

Furthermore, skin resurfacing will not reduce the size of *pores* (except for the "cobblestone" appearance that occurs with rhinophyma). The facial surgeon should explain to the patient that a pore is the surface opening of an oil gland or hair follicle. Attempts to reduce its size may lead to the development of a "pimple."

Resurfacing can sometimes produce a dramatic improvement in the texture of the skin of a patient's face. It may be the best treatment available to the facial surgeon to help obtain a fresher, more youthful skin for the patient. Certainly level II and III resurfacing is not indicated for every patient. It is the facial surgeon's responsibility to determine whether a patient is a candidate for these procedures. A good rule to follow is this: *If in doubt, don't.*

Continued care of a patient's newly resurfaced skin is important to help maintain what has been achieved with the procedures. A professional skin care program administered and overseen by a trained medical aesthetician is recommended.

An effective "selling point" of some *superficial* skin resurfacing technology is that there is no—or limited—"downtime." After 4 decades of performing various levels of skin procedures, by many of the methods available, I have come to the following conclusion: the downside of no downtime is that there are also no—or very limited—long-term results.

The following discussion is shared with patients *prior to skin resurfacing,* and reinforced at every opportunity during the posttreatment period.

Healing occurs in stages. The length of time required for any treated area to heal varies from one individual to the other and from one procedure/treatment to the other. The patient's adherence to the surgeon's instructions and admonitions plays a vital role in how quickly—and well—a treated part of the human body heals.

Some degree of swelling follows any surgical procedure. The swelling is due to the new tissue fluids brought into the area by the body to promote healing. The increased blood supply to the region is responsible for the pink color of the skin and some of the irregular coloration associated with level II and III procedures. When these healing fluids are no longer required, the tissues release them and they are absorbed through the bloodstream.

A patient must be willing to accept the swelling and discoloration that occurs following such operations. Though these natural sequelae are usually visually disconcerting, most people feel they are a negligible inconvenience to pay for the physical and psychological improvement they generally experience.

The surgeon must not fail to ask patients if they have taken Accutane (Roche, New York, NY). It is generally recommended that none of the resurfacing procedures discussed in this chapter be performed for at least 12 months after discontinuing Accutane.

Resurfaced skin may display differences in coloration after skin resurfacing. Melanocytes are found in the deeper layers of the dermis. A rule of thumb is that superficial resurfacing procedures tend to stimulate the growth of melanocytes, thereby creating hyperpigmentation, whereas deeper (level III) resurfacing procedures destroy melanocytes and produce hypopigmentation. However, I have performed many dermabrasions on patients with African ancestry. Initially all pigment is removed. Within a couple of weeks it begins to return. Whereas Caucasian skin is pink in the early stages of healing, patients with black skin notice that the skin is darker. Within months the darker shades fade.

In patients with all ethnic backgrounds, should hyperpigmentation persist, it can be bleached with combination therapy of Retin-A and hydroquinone. Some experts suggest limiting the use of hydroquinone to 3-month intervals.

■ Reference

1. McCollough, EG, Langsdon, PR. Dermabrasion and Chemical Peel: A Guide for Facial Plastic Surgeons. New York, NY: Thieme Medical Pub. 1988

22 Chemical Peeling

A chemical peel involves the careful application of a scientifically formulated solution to the skin, which later causes the top layer to separate and shed (as would a blister) (**Fig. 22.1**). The shedding skin takes with it the sun-damaged and wrinkled layers. Swelling of the peeled area may be pronounced for the first few days but subsides dramatically after 5 to 7 days.

Level II and III peels heal as would a sunburn or a blister, in that the top layer of skin is shed or "peels off" over a 4- to 5-day period, revealing the early signs of a fresh new deep pink layer underneath.

Depending on the level of the peel, *mineral powder makeup* may be used approximately 3 weeks after the application of the peeling solution; therefore, most patients may return to work or go out socially at this time. When instructions and precautions are heeded by the patient, the redness of the skin slowly subsides over the ensuing 6 to 8 weeks, but it can ordinarily be camouflaged by makeup during this time. However, in patients who fail to follow directions, it may take months before deep pink or reddish discoloration subsides. In every case, I have been able to *eventually* get to the root of the problem. Fact is, many patients are reluctant to admit that they used products or engaged in activities advised against.

Limitations and Restrictions

Avoidance of *prolonged* exposure to sunlight (as in sunbathing, fishing, and golfing) for 3 to 6 months and of skin irritants are fundamental restrictions after peeling. The "new" skin must build up a tolerance to the elements; otherwise, healing is delayed. Patients who fail to adhere to instructions and precautions may develop pigmentation, skin irritations—and in rare cases—scarring.

All patients contemplating level II and level III peels must be willing to accept the posttreatment restrictions required to promote healing.

Patients must also be informed that *neither surgery nor resurfacing can correct wrinkles that occur only during facial expressions.* Creases around the eyes produced by smiling, the forehead creases that occur with frowning, and the vertical lines in the upper lip that occur with puckering the lips for the most

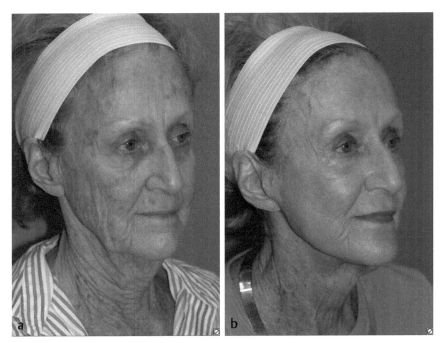

Fig. 22.1   **(a)** Prior to a chemical peel. **(b)** After the chemical peel.

part are due to the contraction of the muscles of facial expression. *None* of the *surgical procedures* discussed in this book are able to eliminate the preceding conditions. However, neuromodulators can be helpful in treating these conditions.

If wrinkles and creases are present with the face *at rest,* then resurfacing combined with surgery may improve them.

Patients are often misinformed about the long-term restriction of activities following a peel or dermabrasion. They have heard that once they have had a peel (or dermabrasion) they can *never* get in the sun again—this, too, has not been my experience.

While it is important to avoid sun exposure and to use sunscreen products for the first 6 months, ordinary sun exposure after that is strongly recommended. It simply takes time for the new skin to toughen or build up a natural resistance to sun and wind.

23 Dermabrasion

When the skin has an irregular or uneven texture from acne scarring or from previous injuries, a level II or III dermabrasion (performed with a spinning brush or fraise) may provide improvement. It is also a helpful adjunct to laser resurfacing when treating wrinkled, sun-damaged, or deeply pigmented areas of skin (**Fig. 23.1**).

The technique of dermabrasion is equivalent to sanding a scratch from a wooden surface in that the work is actually done on the *elevated areas* in an attempt to take them down closer to the lowest portion of the defect. When successful, this diminishes the high–low junctions that are responsible for casting shadows when light strikes the face from an angle. The result is skin that is smoother and tighter than before.

When the texture of the facial skin is very irregular from excessive or deep scarring, a second treatment may be required 6 to 12 months after the initial treatment. These drawings represent an area of skin that might contain scars and defects of different widths, depths, and configurations (**Fig. 23.2**).

As the drawings demonstrate, the more superficial defects might be completely removed by dermabrasion. Those that are moderately deep may be improved but not removed, and some of the deeper or "ice-pick" type scars may not be improved at all.

In some cases a *second* dermabrasion within 6 to 12 months can provide additional improvement to those moderately deep scars (**Fig. 23.3, Fig. 23.4**). In some circumstances, dermabrasion can be done a third time, but there is a limit. Prior to surgery it is difficult to predict the degree of improvement, since each patient's skin responds to the same treatment by the same surgeon in a different manner.

Skin pores are the surface openings of the oil glands. Neither dermabrasion, nor a laser, nor a peel is designed to alter them.

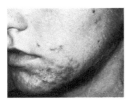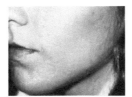

Fig. 23.1   When cystic acne does not respond to medical treatment, a level III therapeutic dermabrasion can often improve both the appearance and medical problems in the affected areas. The procedure may be repeated if necessary within several months. Although I do not contend that dermabrasion is a treatment for every case of acne, many patients have received some improvement following this procedure. Acne is generally a medical condition, not surgical; therefore, its treatment should be supervised by the patient's dermatologist.

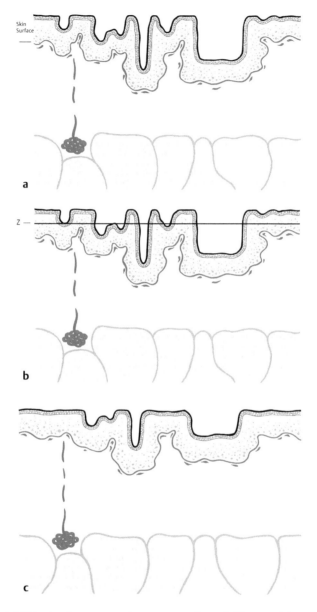

Fig. 23.2 **(a)** This drawing represents a cross-section of skin containing a variety of defects. The defects may vary in depth, width, and configuration. Some are very deep, penetrating far down into the dermis. **(b)** Dermabrasion (at level Z) generally removes the epidermal (top) layer of skin. Many of the more superficial defects may be completely eliminated, and those of intermediate depth improved, but the deeper ones are only slightly better. **(c)** After a level III dermabrasion, a new layer of skin forms at a lower level. **(d)** Often a second dermabrasion (at level Z) can be performed within another 6- to 12-month period. **(e)** Following two level II or III procedures, some defects still exist, but one may see improvement in the overall texture and consistency of the skin.

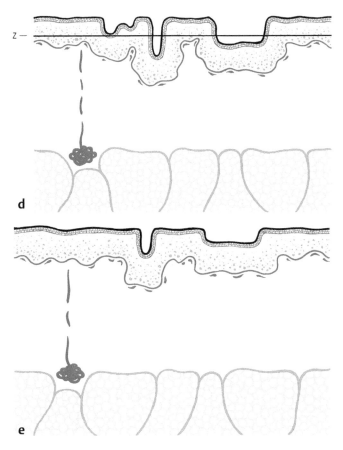

Fig. 23.2 **(d)** Often a second dermabrasion (at level Z) can be performed within another 6- to 12-month period. **(e)** Following two level II or III procedures, some defects still exist, but one may see improvement in the overall texture and consistency of the skin.

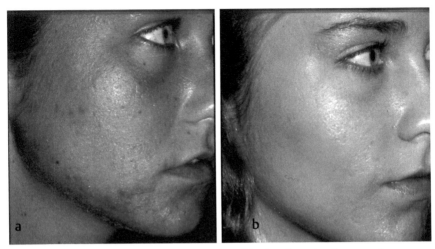

Fig. 23.3   (a) Prior to a dermabrasion procedure. (b) After dermabrasion procedure.

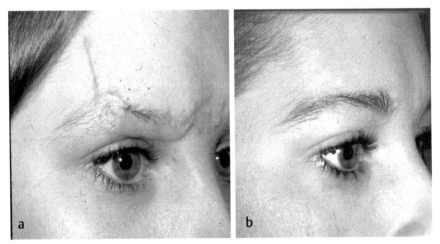

Fig. 23.4   (a) Prior to a scar revision and dermabrasion procedure. (b) After scar revision and two dermabrasion procedures.

24 Laser Surgery

All lasers are not the same. They are tools or instruments that come in a variety of different forms and are designed to perform different tasks. Some lasers vaporize the outer layers of sun-damaged or aging skin. Some can also pass through the outer layers of the skin and destroy deeper birthmarks (port-wine stains) or tiny blood vessels (spider veins.)

As is the case with most technology, the use of lasers is an art form that improves with training and experience. Lasers, like any technology, must be used for the right reasons. The right reason is that, in the facial surgeon's opinion, it is superior to other forms of treatment, in terms of safety and outcomes. For some conditions, lasers exceed other forms of treatment. For others, I have found laser therapies to be inferior. So, if training in dermabrasion and chemical peeling was not offered during residency or fellowship, it is recommended that the surgeon arrange to spend enough time with a colleague who performs these procedures to feel comfortable offering and performing them.

Information about skin resurfacing technology is best received from experienced surgical colleagues, *not from the sales representatives of the companies who manufacture and sell the equipment.* And keep in mind that some colleagues are compensated spokespersons for technology companies. When reading written materials or attending lectures on skin resurfacing, pay attention to disclosures each speaker is required to state at the beginning of the presentation.

■ Laser Hair Removal

Unwanted hair on various parts of the body haunts men and women. Fortunately, there are lasers that can address the problem, when the hair is dark. Fine, lightly colored hair is more difficult to eradicate. Laser therapy will remove existing hairs. Those that have not yet come through the skin may require some future treatment.

Most treatment protocols usually take three to six treatments to be effective, spaced every 6 to 8 weeks. After these treatments most patients have no growth of hair for a period of time. That time may vary from months to years.

In reality, "laser hair removal" should be considered "hair reduction" because a small percentage of hair grows back, no matter what form of laser hair removal is used. And patients should be thusly informed *prior to treatment*. Patients who experience regrowth of hair, however, will usually have a finer, less dense population of hair in that anatomical area. Electrolysis and other spa treatments may achieve additional improvement.

Laser-assisted hair removal is less painful and provides longer-lasting results than the traditional methods of hair removal (electrolysis). In experienced hands, scarring is much less apt to occur with laser hair removal than with electrolysis.

Laser hair removal has several advantages. In experienced hands, it is a safe and cost-effective method with few side effects. This method takes a matter of minutes and is virtually pain free. It is also the most effective method of permanent hair reduction *approved by the U.S. Food and Drug Administration (FDA)*.

■ Dilated Blood Vessels, Rosacea, and Pigmented Spots

After years of unprotected sun exposure, the skin will lose its smooth, uniform, youthful appearance. Certain chronic skin conditions (like rosacea) can also cause damage to the collagen and elastic fibers of the dermal layers. Maintenance and rejuvenation of collagen and elastic fibers help maintain a youthful appearance to the skin. Some types of skin conditions improved by laser therapy are benign vascular lesions (telangiectasias, rosacea, flushing, hemangiomas), sunspots, photoaging, different colorations in the skin, fine wrinkles, large pores, and loss of tone and elasticity.

■ Leg Veins

Different types of lasers are used to address various kinds of vascular lesions (Fig. 24.1).

Among these lesions are included problematic leg vessels. These superficial vascular problems include small spider veins and larger varicose veins. Traditionally, sclerotherapy (concentrated salt solution) and surgical intervention with stripping were the main methods of treatment for patients with this problem. Advantages of laser therapy are a lower rate of side effects, shorter healing time, and the absence of compression therapy after treatment when compared with traditional therapy.

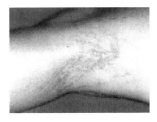

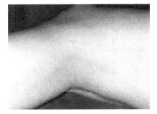

Fig. 24.1   Dilated veins and capillaries.

■ Acne

Acne affects about 80% of the human population. It is caused by the obstruction, inflammation, and infection of the oil glands of the skin. This condition normally presents itself during the adolescent years due to the hormonal changes in the body's oil glands during this time that cause them to become occluded. However, it can occur in adults as well.

Different modalities of medical treatments for acne have been tried. Unfortunately, many patients fail to respond to them, including topical or systemic antibiotics, Accutane (Roche, New York, NY) therapy, and hundreds of over-the-counter remedies.

Lasers and intense pulsed light (IPL) have been shown to improve acne in many patients, with few side effects; however, it may require as many as eight treatments over a period of 4 weeks. In resistant cases it may be necessary to work with a dermatologist to provide the maximum degree of improvement.

25 Injectable Therapies: Botox, Fillers, Fat, and Fascia

In recent years, nonsurgical techniques and devices for rejuvenating the aging face have taken the profession by storm.

It is my firm conviction that most of the more dramatic, meaningful, natural, favorable—and in the long run, *economical*—examples of facial rejuvenation are accomplished through the expert application of *time-honored surgical techniques*. In my experience the use of fascia or scar harvested from the patient's own body has proven to be the most economical and long-lasting method of filling thinning lips and deep facial grooves. Fat is less predictable, and the vast majority of commercial fillers provide only temporary improvement.

Neuromodulators, fat, and fillers can be used in some patients who wish to lessen lines and wrinkles created by facial expression. Many younger adults choose to use neuromodulators in an attempt to slow the development of the undesirable signs of aging. It is my opinion that *all options* should be discussed with patients, even if the patient requests a certain product. Doing so fulfills the physician's requirement for "informed consent."

Neuromodulators have gained popularity and can be used for a variety of facial issues. These injections can lessen expression wrinkles about the forehead and crow's-feet area. I have reservations about using neuromodulators in the peri-oral region of the face, except when extreme puckering of the mentalis muscle occurs with facial expression. The temporary paralysis with neuromodulators is different than what is accomplished with skin resurfacing. In some cases a combination of neuromodulators *and* resurfacing is recommended.

Neuromodulators may also be injected to improve some of the spasms and asymmetry that patients with facial paralysis and Bell's palsy experience. It should be noted that results obtained with neuromodulators are not permanent, so their use will have to be repeated. And undesirable lagophthalmos (ptosis) of the upper eyelid has been reported, as well as drooping of the upper lip and drooling at the corners of the mouth.

Much attention is being given to restoring facial volume with a variety of synthetic materials. Commercially available "fillers" have become one of the most popular cosmetic procedures in the industry. Most are short-lived and require repeated injections every several months. This is not the venue to discuss specific commercial products, only to urge facial surgeons to investigate the claims made by the company and ask for independent histological proof that a product does what it claims to do.

Soft tissue grafts have long been used in plastic surgery. The first breast augmentations were en bloc fat grafts, but because hard lumps (healed areas of fat necrosis) made it difficult to distinguish scar from cancer, the practice was abandoned.

Fat harvested from other parts of the body has been injected into various regions of the body. It appears that the skill of the surgeon in harvesting the graft and preparing it for reinjection and the skill with which the fat cells are injected are the keys to success. Still, many surgeons are beginning to reveal that varying degrees of injected fat remains and retreatment is usually necessary. A rule of thumb is this: *fat injected into muscle tends to survive more often than fat cells injected into fat or subcutaneous tissues.*

I recommend that anyone who plans to incorporate fat grafting into their practice spend an appropriate amount of time with an experienced surgeon who has performed hundreds—if not thousands—of fat grafts, and learn the finer details of the procedure.

For the past 15 years I have used en bloc grafts composed of fat and fascia in the face. The most common source of these grafts is the preparotid fat and fascia of the superficial musculoaponeurotic system (SMAS), obtained at the time of facelift surgery (**Fig. 25.1**).

The second most available sites are the postauricular sulcus and preoccipital fascia. In cases where a facelift is not performed, a source of fascia is the postauricular region. While there is less fat available, the collagenous fascia in these areas is usually more abundant. A scar from a previous injury or surgery makes the most ideal of all "filler" grafts. It is necessary, however, to remove the skin overlying the deeper scar tissue.

In my experience, the success rate for fascia/fat en bloc grafting has been high. It is used to augment thinning lips, melolabial grooves, and deep glabellar lines (**Fig. 25.2**).

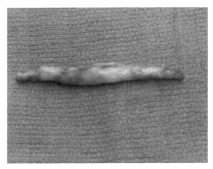

Fig. 25.1 Strip of SMAS and fat obtained during facelifting surgery.

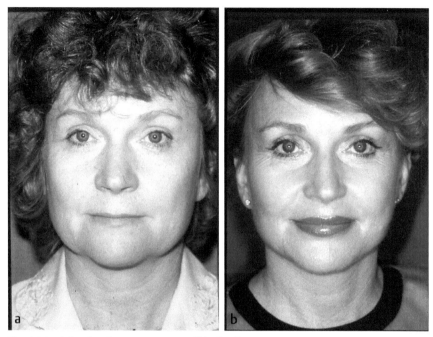

Fig. 25.2 **(a)** Before lip augmentation. **(b)** After lip augmentation.

When one calculates the costs of temporary fillers for a period of 3 to 5 years, they often exceed the cost of surgery. With surgery *some* improvement will be visible forever. With temporary fillers, once the last molecule has been broken down by the body, the patient has nothing to show for the money.

As is the case with any facial volumizing technique, the key is to avoid over-treatment. A face that appears "overvolumized" and does not exhibit the natural junction contours between anatomical regions—or in which features are unproportionally volumized—loses the "natural" appearance that can be achieved by well-performed facial plastic surgery. Appearing "plastic" is one of the most commonly expressed concerns I hear from patients contemplating appearance-enhancing surgery. Yet the same can be said about injudicious use of injectable fillers. The facial surgeon who can allay these fears will attract a greater percentage of the population.

IV The Administrative and Risk Management Side of a Facial Surgery Practice

26 The Right Facial Surgery Practice Model

No one-size-fits-all practice model for facial surgeons exists. The option you select should be based upon several factors. First, you must decide if you intend to be recognized as a facial surgeon or someone whose core specialty practice *also* includes facial surgery. In making that determination, there are three cardinal questions to be considered:

- Are you an independent thinker—an entrepreneur?
- Are you more comfortable working in a team environment?
- Do you prefer to have the backing of a large institution behind you and an academic title?

How these questions are answered should direct you toward a particular style of practice.

- The entrepreneur will likely lean toward solo practice in a private setting.
- The team player will likely be attracted to a group practice or partnership.
- And the institutionalist will likely be intrigued by joining the full-time faculty of a university, large multispecialty clinic, or hospital.

Regardless of which route you choose, you should surround yourself with a team of advisors and counselors: an attorney, an accountant, and a financial advisor.

From that team, you will likely be advised to create a corporate structure under which you will conduct your practice. In today's times, the limited liability company (LLC) serves the needs of most physicians. However, such laws vary from state to state. You should sign any contractual practice agreement as the "managing member" of the LLC you and your attorney create.

A corporate veil protects accumulated assets against legal judgments without the necessity of working under a potentially onerous board of directors. In addition, the tax savings advantages of an LLC avoid the double taxation that some other corporate structures (C corporation) require. Your attorney and accountant will advise you as to the appropriate course of action. They will also be in a position to recommend banks in your area that solicit business relationships with physicians.

If you conduct business as an LLC, lending and financing institutions will likely require "personal guarantees" to ensure that monies owed will be paid.

If you are inclined to practice in a group or institutional practice (ranging from 1 to 100 associates), you should carefully examine the professional (and personal) image and character of each and every associate. Throughout your career, the venerable axiom *"you are known by the company you keep"* will be an asset, or an albatross. During due diligence investigation, learn about the "significant other" of each associate. Determine whose mind-set you will be dealing with on a daily basis—the physician associate, or the associate's significant other. Determine who "wears the pants" in the household. Significant others implode a professional relationship between collegial physicians more often than you might imagine.

You should enter your professional career with the knowledge that doctors are trained to be independent thinkers and that compliance to policies, procedures, and protocols created *by others* is often resisted.

Perhaps the ideal practice opportunity for someone just entering practice is to find an aesthetic surgeon who primarily specializes in body plastic surgery and offer expertise in facial aesthetic surgery to that practice.

The next best scenario is to find an established facial surgeon who is contemplating retirement. Win that surgeon's confidence and enter into a long-term contract to continue the practice. The wise young associate will readily adapt to the same policies and procedures that made the practice successful in the first place. History affirms that when a young surgeon takes over the practice of a long-standing icon and begins to make changes, patients seek the kind of care they experienced from the senior surgeon elsewhere. Too many "assumed" practices fail because the new owner "fixed" what was not broken.

Building a private solo practice should be viewed as a 5-year project. Joining a group or institution can shorten the curve. However, long-term returns generally fall to physicians who build their own practice (within the larger practice) and own (at least, in part) the office/clinic in which the practice operates.

Initial contracts of 1 to 2 years are recommended. That gives both the new surgeon and the partners an opportunity to see if the arrangement should be extended. If it becomes clear that you are not the right "fit" for the practice you join, it is best to end the relationship as soon as possible. No physician should have to deal with interprofessional dissension at work.

27 Practice Theory Put into Practice Action

The following testimonials are shared so that readers may see how the policies, procedures, and protocols in this book can actually be applied to the evolving practice of a young facial plastic surgeon. As I (their fellowship director) recommended, each of the physicians whose stories I share chose to limit their practice to facial plastic surgery, from the outset.

First we hear from Dr. Marshall Guy, who established a solo private practice in the Highlands community, just outside Houston, Texas:

> I had the pleasure of completing a facial plastic and reconstructive surgery fellowship with Dr. McCollough from July 2014 until June 2015. In addition to the amazing surgical training, I was able to get much-appreciated advice on how to open my own business, as I planned on starting my own private practice. Since he had successfully opened practices at least three times over his career, I knew he would be a treasure trove of information.
>
> I can remember the long car ride we went on together for a meeting, where I had the chance to pick his brain for his advice. After we returned from that event, I wrote down nearly two pages of notes on what we had discussed. I am glad I did this because I still refer back to those notes now as my business continues to grow. And although times have changed since he opened his most −recent office location, the advice is still very much applicable.
>
> Using his recommendations has helped my new facial plastic surgery office grow quickly and reach profitability much faster than I had anticipated. Throughout this book I am sure you will learn many of these tidbits, but I have elected to share a few of them now.
>
> The recommendation I remember hearing over and over again is be a facial plastic surgeon. If this is what you truly want to do, then this is what you need to do. I am very proud of my otolaryngology training and the skills that I developed there to help make me a better surgeon, but if you go out and become an otolaryngologist

and facial plastic surgeon, you will inevitably be an otolaryngologist and do very little facial plastic surgery.

With a new office where every patient counts, turning away general otolaryngology patients was certainly not easy. But I have found this statement to be so true. As a facial specialist in an area with over 20 plastic surgeons and three other fellowship-trained facial plastic surgeons, as the only one exclusively practicing facial plastic surgery, I have had numerous patients indicate that is why they came to me. They wanted a facial specialist. That is hard advice to follow in the beginning, but well worth it if you want your practice to be facial plastic and reconstructive surgery.

The second recommendation made to me by Dr. McCollough is one I'd like to share. *Go where everyone else is.* Open up shop across the street from the busiest plastic surgeons and facial plastic surgeons in town. People associate that area with aesthetics. They expect to get cosmetic surgery when they are there. There is a reason that people haven't set up shop in certain areas, so don't go set up shop in those areas. At first, Dr. McCollough's advice seemed counterintuitive, as I felt it would be nice to be the only one somewhere. But that doesn't usually work because all the people who came before you already looked at that area and that market didn't work. By being where everyone else is, you will get plenty of patients.

The final recommendation Dr. McCollough made to me relates to overhead (the cost of doing business). I found a space I liked and could afford that is right across the street from one of the busiest plastic surgeons in my area. I was approached by every device manufacturer and skin care company to buy their products and machines. They all make great pitches. But what distinguishes us from others who perform aesthetic services is *our surgical ability*, which we bring to our practice with no overhead (other than the loans it took to reach that point in our training).

Being saddled with another large capital expenditure when you are out on your own can mean the difference between a successful practice and an unsuccessful practice. And most of the expensive devices are more effective when you already have patients to market to instead of getting them in the door in the first place.

I set out on my own in 2015 with the advice provided by Dr. McCollough. And although I have had to learn some things along the way, using his guidance and recommendations has really made this transition much easier and more enjoyable.

Social marketing is really the lifeblood of a new practice. For those who are more established, it helps to keep patients and recruit more. But for those who are just opening their facial plastic surgery practice, it is an absolute must.

The questions arise how, what, and where to engage in social marketing. Unfortunately, there is no magic bullet that works for everyone, and in different markets different media will be more effective. The largest social media network is going to be Facebook. At the least your business needs a Facebook page. This should not be designed simply as a brochure, but as a way to engage your audience. You or a member of your marketing team needs to post something at least weekly to keep your audience entertained. This may be answers to commonly asked questions, discussing new technologies or treatments, or simply providing general tips to help keep your clients looking their best. The key is consistency so people know to look for your post.

When it comes to Facebook, you will need to build your audience. This can be accomplished organically (meaning you didn't pay for it), but sharing your professional page with all of your friends is a quick way to get some likes. When your friends see your posts they can like them and also share them, which then leads to a blossoming effect for views. The other way to get likes and visualization of your post is to pay for it. This is faster and easier, but it costs money. You can also highly select the audience that you want based on demographics, although this does add to the cost of marketing. Once you have the likes, you can then begin marketing to people who have already liked your page. This focuses your dollars on those already interested in your services, which makes the return on investment higher.

In addition to Facebook, Twitter is another medium for social marketing. Twitter is a microblogging site that allows you to send out messages to your followers. To keep your audience engaged, you really need to be putting out tweets more frequently than your Facebook posts. This should be daily if possible. It is a nice medium for getting out information quickly to your followers. Unlike Facebook, where your posts may or may not be seen by your audience, your tweets will go out to all of your followers. Whether they read them or not is up to them, but they can at least see that you sent them out.

The last social medium I wanted to comment on is Instagram. Being that our field is visual, this can be a great source of marketing. It does carry with it the most liability to make sure you are HIPAA compliant, but it is a great way for your followers to post about their experience with you (when the patient is posting, it is not breaking HIPAA, but double-check with your legal team).

Because your patients can see you in your photos, it is a great way to keep people engaged.

Finally, on your own Web site you can include a blog. This is a great way to keep all of your Facebook posts, tweets, and photos in one place. There are also services that can automatically populate each of your social media posts for you (so you can have one post or announcement that goes to all of them and is also archived on your blog).

The key with all of this is content. Making original content is ideal because it separates you from the pack. Anyone can pay a marketing company to post canned items. This will not improve your rankings on search engines, but it is one way of delegating the social media aspect. But if you really want to engage your audience, write the posts yourself. The great thing is you can write a lot of posts ahead of time and schedule them. See Chapter 5 for details.

(W. Marshall Guy, MD, Facial Plastic and Reconstructive Surgeon, Woodlands, Texas)

Next I share the experience of Dr. Parker A. Velargo, a facial plastic surgeon and former fellow, who established a practice with a long-time friend who specialized in comprehensive plastic surgery. Both doctors entered practice straight out of their training and formed a partnership in New Orleans, Louisiana.

I distinctly remember my first time interacting with Dr. McCollough at his massive, well-run clinic in Gulf Shores, Alabama. It was the day I interviewed for a fellowship with one of the giants in our field of facial plastic surgery. After a day of watching him perform surgery and interact with his patients during consultations and follow-up appointments, we had a discussion about my future plans. His advice was simple—come here and I'll give you all the tools you need to have a successful and thriving practice.

One year later, I joined Dr. McCollough as his fellow for a year, and I can attest that I would not be as successful as I am right now without learning a great deal from this man. While I cannot consolidate all that I have learned in this testimonial to Dr. McCollough's knowledge on preparing to enter practice and marketing, I can comment on several things.

There is no better tool for preparing to enter a private practice in facial plastic surgery than your knowledge and skills. Thus, I absorbed as much as I could from Dr. McCollough during my fellowship. I learned how to interact with patients, how to manage complications, how to manage "difficult" patients, how to perform consultations in a manner that reduced patient anxiety and increased surgical conversion. Of course I learned how to operate, but more importantly, I learned how to run an efficient and organized operating room (OR). I learned what I could realistically expect from my future staff because I saw the gold standard. I learned how to train assistants for optimal clinic and surgical efficiency. I learned the importance of patient education. I learned more than I can type here, but it's this knowledge that set the foundation for the way that I run my practice currently and the future direction I want to take it.

Perhaps the single most effective marketing practice I learned from Dr. McCollough was to "get out of the office." It's tempting to perform a great deal of facial plastic surgery procedures in one's clinic procedure room; however, nobody knows you when you are starting out.

Dr. McCollough's advice to get out of the office and operate on patients in surgery centers and hospitals has proven to be a valuable referral source for me. When the staff at these facilities see the work that you do and get to know you on a personal basis, your reputation in the community grows. One lesson that came from pure observation was that Dr. McCollough was never afraid to "hire out" for certain tasks if his time was more valuable elsewhere.

Even though I have a fairly young practice and cannot afford to "hire out" as much as I desire, this holds true for a very important example for me—building and managing a Web site and search engine optimization (SEO). I pay a nominal fee on a monthly basis for a company to manage my Web site, blog for my practice, post on several social media outlets, and organically drive up my SEO. In my opinion, the specifics of these essential marketing practices do not need to be self-taught.

A single facelift more than covers the cost of what is paid annually for these services. And, such services, when provided by a professional company, will actually drive more patients to you. So, spending my time where I can provide the most for my practice is an essential lesson learned during my fellowship.

Lastly, I will comment on the concept of "practice patience." Facial plastic surgeons face a unique situation because the general population does not understand our training background. While it is perfectly acceptable for a comprehensive plastic surgeon to perform hand surgery to generate extra income in the early stages of their career, facial plastic surgeons who perform general ears, nose, and throat (ENT) procedures will not be viewed as favorably in the community.

Maintaining a good reputation in the community as an excellent facial plastic surgeon requires "practice patience"—it takes 2 to 5 years for a private facial plastic surgery practice to become steadily busy.

However, when faced with a lower than desired income out of the gate and pressure from a spouse who has waited over 10 years for you to "make it," it is tempting to become shortsighted and start practicing general ENT to supplement your income. The community then views you as an ENT doctor who does some facial plastic surgery on the side, and the OR staff, as well as the community, no longer view you as an expert in facial plastic surgery. I have seen this firsthand in my community, and this issue was stressed by Dr. McCollough throughout my training.

Having trained nearly 100 fellows, he has seen some fellows fall into this trap and knows what the outcome always is. So, "practice patience" builds reputation, which in turn leads to long-term success with endless possibilities.

Dr. McCollough's length of time in private practice is an asset to contributing to a book on starting a practice. While the digital age and securing funds to start a practice have certainly evolved over time, these are easy things to figure out along the way.

Dr. McCollough's advice takes into account all of the mistakes and successes that he has made along the way and all of the things that have failed him and worked for him over the years—what better way to start a practice than learning from this unparalleled experience?

(Parker A. Velargo, MD,

New Orleans Center for Aesthetics and Plastic Surgery)

These two outstanding young facial surgeons exemplify what is possible, providing many of the policies, procedures, and protocols herein recommended are followed. They are a compilation of my experience, as well as that of my mentors, Drs. Jack R. Anderson, Richard Webster, and Walter E. Berman.

Hopefully, sharing the preceding experiences will provide "food for thought" to the surgeon contemplating fellowship training in aesthetic and reconstructive facial surgery.

28 The Practice as an Investment

Over their career facial surgeons will generate a lot of money. Whether they *accumulate wealth* is another matter. This chapter is intended to provide guidance on money management and fiscal responsibility, both within the practice and in one's personal life.

◼ A Stereotype to Be Overcome

In "Why Doctors Can't Manage Money," investopedia.com noted, "Doctors are one of our most esteemed professions. They're held up as geniuses, seemingly unable to do wrong. Except when it comes to money."

The fact that doctors are not looked upon as good managers of their affairs makes us targets to industries that prey on the medical profession's lack of business training. Physicians are usually so busy taking care of patients and practicing defensive medicine that we don't always pay attention to financial matters, at least not until we learn by being burned. Hopefully, this chapter will go a long way in helping you avoid being indoctrinated by fire.

The Investopedia article goes on to say, "A common stereotype [is that] doctors...rack up debt, spend too much of their income and fail to save for retirement."[1]

In the same article, Dr. Jim Dahle contends that the stereotype stems from "a lack of financial literacy, poor financial discipline and a lack of long-term perspective. In addition," he said, "there is a bit of a culture within academic medicine where you don't talk about financial topics."[2]

As is the case with most issues, balance is the key—knowing when to spend, knowing when to save, knowing when to invest, and into what. This chapter emphasises the wisdom of investing in one's practice.

In addition to his academic responsibilities, the chairman of my residency program managed a very successful private practice. Thankfully, he did not hesitate to share financial matters with his residents. The following is one of the "secrets" he shared: "The doctor who brags about a low overhead could be penny wise and pound foolish."

Dr. Hicks was referring to the fact that a surgeon should not skimp on essentials necessary to be productive and accommodating. Good business practices call for surrounding oneself with a competent staff. This includes medical and paramedical personnel, to whom the surgeon can delegate tasks such as prescreening patients, assessing laboratory tests, application and removal of dressings, and basic wound and skin care.

The other part of the equation is to know when enough is enough. For more advice on this matter, I recommend the book *Parkinson's Law*.[3] It is a brilliant dissertation by Dr. C. Northcote Parkinson, a 20th-century British economist. His law states, "Work expands to fill the time available for its completion." To this, I add, "Work is not necessarily synonymous with productivity." I include another corollary to Dr. Parkinson's law: Being present is not necessarily working. Work is measurable, either in profits or in reduction of stress for the owner/manager of the practice. If an employee or associate is not rising to either of these criteria, that employee is a drag on the practice.

■ The Office Makes a Statement

In Chapter 3, I discussed the strategic location of one's practice. That includes the assistance of an architect schooled in the design of medical/surgical facilities and a professional interior designer. Their charge must be to design and decorate the facility with tasteful décor that creates an inviting ambiance and provides the considerate privacy expected of an elite facial surgery practice. The elite facial surgery clinic is careful not to offend anyone who enters the door. Extravagance is not only unnecessary; it can be interpreted as poor taste. In that regard, a visitor should not be faced with anything that they might find offensive, for example, school colors and memorabilia of the surgeon's favorite sports team. And the practice setting need not be expansive to impress.

■ On the Matter of Compromise

Many young doctors enter practice with large debts hanging over their heads, usually in the form of "student loans." Debt often forces compromise and limits opportunity. Though they may not be the best option for building an elite practice, practice settings in which income and benefits are guaranteed appear more attractive. In these cases, the surgeon is often required to provide services that are not related to aesthetic facial surgery. The public perceives *any doctor* who performs plastic surgery to be a "plastic surgeon," regardless of the parameters that exist within the medical profession. And surgeons who perform services outside the facial region will find it more difficult to establish themselves as a "facial surgeon." The bottom line is this: the sooner one dedicates oneself to facial surgery, the sooner one will be on the way to establishing an elite facial surgery practice.

■ The Facial Surgeon's Consulting Team

An elite facial surgery practice should have an elite team of trusted consultants. It is never a bad idea to check with the local Better Business Bureau, state bar, and accountancy and financial planning oversight board to see if the consultant you are considering is in "good standing." You should also ask for references of other clients represented by the consultant. And follow up by speaking directly to several of the references provided. It is also a good practice to ask for references *outside* the medical profession. And do not limit background checks to one's consulting team. It is a good idea to check on anyone you hire. There is a reason I began this chapter with the stereotype assigned to us physicians.

While you will want to contact business individuals outside the medical profession, make sure the attorney and accountant you hire are experienced in dealing with issues that pertain to medical practices. A facial surgeon needs a consultant who knows about a "fee for service" business model.

As indicated with the décor of the practice, a facial surgeon should exercise prudence when hiring consultants. Accountants and attorneys charge *for their time*, including research and preparation for meetings, usually in 20-minute increments. A facial surgeon might not always get the best advice from the most expensive consultant. You should know what each increment costs; and keep a diary of when you consult with each advisor. Subtly, let the consultant know that you are doing so. One way to do so is to ask, when did we "go on the clock?" And in the case of face-to-face meetings, write the answer down, in front of the advisor.

During the interview process, you should also insist that anytime the consultant's fee schedule changes, you are to be notified at least 30 days in advance. "Memorandums of understanding" specify contractual agreements between the facial surgeon and each consultant.

Here, I share the advice of my Scotch-Irish father—a man reared on a dirt farm during the Great Depression of the early 20th century. He was only able to obtain an eighth-grade education in a one-room schoolhouse. Yet along the road of life, a member of what journalist Tom Brokow called America's "greatest generation,"[4] my father acquired the wisdom of the ages. As though it were yesterday, I recall the day he said to me, "In some cases, saving money is as profitable as—or better than—earning it. You may not be required to pay taxes on money saved."

Some financial advisors ask for an annual retainer, plus commissions on transactions they conduct on your behalf. In keeping with the costly principle I label "learn by being burned," I learned to ask—sooner, rather than later—about the billing practices of every member of a surgeon's consulting team. Doing so can save you money and consternation. Fortunately, I discovered the commission game in time to take corrective action.

It is a sad state of affairs that you as a doctor have to view—with some degree of skepticism—those hired to look after your interests. Scandals within the investment industry are documented facts. As one goes through life, one lesson remains constant, that there are people who will sell their souls for money and power, regardless of the titles that might precede and follow their names.

I share my own experiences to encourage you to pay attention to the business practices of those you should be able to trust. Assume nothing. Ask about hidden fees. Use the time you spend with consultants wisely. Then, insist on an e-mail report about the decisions reached during all meetings, including telephone calls. In my practice, I tell my staff, "Assume that a telephone call never happened. In the case of a dispute, it is one person's word against the other's." Add the e-mail to the file you create for *each consultant,* just in case.

Based upon experience, I advise against retainers for consulting services. Insist that the invoice you receive from a hired consultant be itemized with the *exact time billed*, who performed the service, and the amount assigned to each firm member. Review the invoice for accuracy before you pay. And do not hesitate to question the bill if you feel that it does not accurately reflect the time for which you are being billed.

Many large law and accounting firms have billing departments that may have formulas for billing a minimum number of hours for each associate. You should also have the firm document all work performed by the accountant/lawyer, and that of any assistants. Reputable firms will not hesitate to provide full disclosure. If yours does, make the change as soon as possible.

In this chapter, I go one step farther. It is never too early to develop a trusted relationship with a financial planner. You need someone who can provide financial counseling and assist with the prudent management of existing debt and the money you will earn during your career.

■ The Insurance Factor

Do not overlook the importance of insuring the most valuable asset you and your family have—your ability to earn a living. Disability insurance is specifically created for that purpose, should you become disabled. Life insurance is another matter. It provides for your family if you should die. As your children become self-sufficient, the amount of life and disability insurance you need diminishes. Seek outside counsel regarding these matters. The individual selling a given insurance plan is not always the best person to advise you on such matters. You should also ask your financial advisor if they will receive a commission on the insurance plan they recommend, and have them divulge the monetary value of the commission. You are entitled to know such things. If there is hesitation to provide this kind of information, you should consider changing advisors.

Of course you will need "malpractice" insurance. Not having coverage for the doctor is a risk no physician should take—not for a single hour during your career. Choose a company that has a long-standing track record of standing behind its insured physicians, and the doctor's extended staff. And do not skimp on costs here. If your employer provides malpractice coverage, ask to see the policy and have your attorney review it. And know that some behavior is not insured (i.e., altering the medical record, slander and libel).

■ The Equipment and Device Trap

Too many physicians make the fatal mistake of purchasing expensive equipment that could be outdated before it is paid for. Lasers, noninvasive technology claiming to dissolve fat, tighten skin, and remove tattoos or hair, are not only expensive, such machines often do not measure up to claims made.

At a recent facial surgery conference I participated in a panel discussion with several colleagues. The panel addressed advantages of lasers versus chemical peeling or dermabrasion for treating facial rhytids and sun damage. One panel member admitted that before he came to the meeting, he visited the storeroom in his office. There, he estimated that approximately a million dollars' worth of lasers were simply collecting dust. A million dollars is a lot of money. Imagine how that million—wisely invested—could grow into a large retirement "nest egg."

When it comes to equipment, involve your business consultants. Your accountant or tax attorney can present "purchase versus lease" options for tangible assets, such as the machines and technology referenced above. The bottom line is that you should purchase everything you need to build an elite practice, but avoid the temptation to purchase every gadget, device, instrument, or marketing tool or service that are available—or that your competitors have or utilize. Investigate the claims made by technology and services salespersons. Speak directly with colleagues you trust, but look with an element of skepticism if the colleague is a compensated representative (consultant) of the manufacturer. At conferences related to facial surgery, pay attention to "disclosures" of speakers.

When it comes to purchasing equipment and devices, follow the path paved by centuries of wisdom: crawl, walk, run. Lease, when possible. As a rule, the shorter the lease, the better. *Leasing by the day is better than by the year, and so on.* In most states, doctors can find companies that will bring lasers to the doctor's office, along with a technician who can perform some of the procedures scheduled. This requires consolidating patients on certain days, that is, laser days, intense pulsed light (IPL) days, and so on. It is a long-standing tenet of good capitalism: "supply and demand." Start simple. When demand exceeds supply, add what is required. No more; no less.

After returning home from a medical convention or being visited by a sales-person, give yourself a "cooling off" period. Spend a few days assessing whether you must have the "latest and greatest."

It is a fatal—but frequent—mistake to become a slave to one's practice, or whims. By that, I mean consult with your accountant, tax attorney, and financial advisor before purchasing expensive residences, vacation homes, expensive cars, boats, and airplanes. Doctors who spend extravagantly are often compelled to make business and judgment decisions based upon non-business–related financial obligations.

■ Avoiding Financial Ruin

A medical degree is no substitute for good business practices. According to a 2013 article on CNNMoney.com, a disturbing trend over the last few years has been the increasing number of physicians and medical professionals filing for bankruptcy protection. Though many of these bankruptcies are simply Chapter 11 reorganizations, for some bankruptcy sounds the death knell of their prac-tices and careers.

So what is the best way to manage money and prevent financial disaster? The answer is found in an ancient Chinese medical textbook. "Inferior doctors act when conditions are at the end stage; mediocre doctors act early in the course of a condition; superior doctors prevent the condition." It is in the vein of prevention that I share these thoughts on the financial aspects of an elite fa-cial surgery practice.

Wise doctors never stop learning, especially in areas in which they may be lacking. Most medical conventions and conferences offer presentations on practice management. A facial surgeon would be wise to carefully study the program and determine whether attending another lecture on blepharoplasty, facelift surgery, rhinoplasty, or skin resurfacing would be more beneficial than attending a lecture or panel on practice management.

Many colleges and universities allow students (of all ages) to "audit" courses. Early in my practice, I audited a course in business law at the University of Ala-bama at Birmingham (UAB). The auditing option allows one to attend classes (for the usual registration fee), but the attendee is not required to take the examina-tion, and does not receive official credit for taking the course. However, there is no way to assign a monetary value to the things I learned about business law. At the very least, I learned to ask better questions of attorneys and accountants.

■ The Counsel of Business Experts

It is consistent with good business practices to seek counsel from successful businesspeople in one's community. Perhaps the best advice I received as a budding facial surgeon came from a man who owned several automobile dealerships. Like many ultrasuccessful people, he prided himself on mentoring young people. I was one of the fortunate few with whom he shared his formula for success.

"I worked 8 years before I started extracting handsome sums of money out of my businesses," he began. "At the end of each year I invested profits back into my company. I bought another dealership. I only took out enough money for my family and me to live comfortably, in a modest home. Amazingly, after 8 years, it was as though the well (of success) began to overflow," he said. "I wasn't working any harder than the previous 8 years. I wasn't any smarter. I had simply 'primed the pump' until the business took on a life of its own."

Another successful businessman in my community shared advice I have passed on to many young surgeons: "Building a business (practice) is a 5-year plan." The surgeon's spouse must be on board with this part of the plan. After years of living on modest incomes, young families tend to get in a hurry to join the ranks of the (visibly) ultrasuccessful. As a result, they often make financial decisions that make the plan unattainable.

I heeded the counsel of these businessmen. I started small, reinvested profits back into the practice, and owned the real estate on which my practices have been located. Early on, I learned this truism: In 20 years you will have bought a building. If you lease it, you will have bought it for your landlord. If you are your landlord, it is yours to keep, refinance, or sell.

A surgeon can also build equity in the practice itself. In my case, I added aesthetic surgeons to my staff, the majority of whom brought expertise to the practice I either could not offer or chose not to offer (body plastic surgery or reconstructive ophthalmic plastic surgery). However, each also performed some element of facial surgery.

In terms described by the automotive mogul, each associate surgeon became a new "dealership." Once the practice infrastructure is in place it is less costly to add surgeons. And associates can become investors in the practice or the real estate. If the practice continues to flourish, the second-generation surgeons will sell part, or all, of their interests in the practice to the third generation, and so on. This is a sensible way for doctors to build wealth.

A decade and a half after I began the process, I hired a full-time business manager. Together, we created a 60,000–sq ft aesthetic medical center, just up the street from UAB Medical Center in Birmingham, Alabama. The center was a freestanding surgery center with short- and long-term recovery facilities. It offered virtually every service required of an individual striving to look and feel their best—everything from a hair salon, to a medical spa, to nutritional and bariatric medicine—and, of course, aesthetic and reconstructive facial surgery.

The practice and center acquired international recognition, so much so that it was an attractive acquisition for a Wall Street medical enterprise that owned and managed elite medical practices.

To consolidate a series of back and forth negotiations into a very short scenario, an offer was presented that I simply could not refuse. Some payment was offered in stock options. However, the vast majority was a cash offer.

Taking the advice of my business manager, Harold Blach, Jr., and business consultants, I took the deal; I sold the practice, real estate, equipment, and everything. At the age of 52, I had "cashed out." I could have retired. But I chose, instead, to move to a resort community along the Alabama Gulf Coast, where I reinvested a portion of the proceeds. I built a similar—but smaller—version of the Birmingham center, right in the center of an Arnold Palmer–designed golf course resort. And I set the rest of the proceeds aside into a retirement fund for a time when practicing facial surgery might not be an option.

Fortunately, a large percentage of my Birmingham practice followed me to the Gulf Coast. In my new location, I relied on the same principles that made the Birmingham center successful (the ones presented throughout this book). Once again they were instrumental in creating another elite facial surgery practice, this time, within the McCollough Institute for Appearance and Health.

With both ventures, I sought the advice of knowledgeable individuals. I made cautious decisions when the path forward was not clear, and bold moves when the doors of opportunity swung open. Though necessary to preserve the integrity of the practice, some choices were personally painful. As an owner/manager it is sometimes necessary to terminate business relationships.

Once again, I refer to the success model of mentor Coach Paul "Bear" Bryant. When it becomes clear that a team member is acting on advice deemed detrimental to the success of the team (practice), it is time to sever the relationship—*as quickly as possible*. In medical terms, if an infection or cancer is detected, a doctor must not hesitate to take bold action. When other members of the team (practice) witness tolerated insubordination, they begin to lose respect for the manager.

After more than 4 decades of managing a facial surgery practice, I remain committed to the principles that allowed me to create an elite facial surgery practice—and to sharing the things I've learned with as many colleagues as find them helpful.

Once again, my late father was right. When I was a teenager, he said to me, "Son, things are things, and can be lost or taken away. But what you can do with your brain and hands belongs to you for the rest of your life."

So, at age 73, here I am working away, enjoying what I do, with a staff of dedicated associates and employees, in a place that has, rightfully, been called "paradise."

■ The Marden Factor

I conclude this chapter with the counsel of an early 20th century physician and author. In addition to his medical practice, Dr. Orison Swett Marden was the publisher of a widely distributed journal entitled *Success*. To his—and future— generations, Dr. Marden wrote, "The golden opportunity you are seeking is in yourself. It is not in your environment; it is not in luck or chance, or the help of others; it is in yourself alone." The doctor's writings confirmed the advice of a small-town plumber, but a man equally as wise—my father.

As a medical student, I became aware of Dr. Marden's writings, and I have relied upon them to help guide me through the maze of life. On one point, I make deference to the respected expert on success. To build and maintain an elite facial surgery practice, multiple factors must be taken into consideration: Choose the right environment in which to establish one's practice. Choose and train the best people available to assist you. Seek the counsel of ultrasuccessful and honorable people. Then, consider their advice when the doors of opportunity stand before you. Whatever decision you make, know that you weighed the options, then left no room for doubt.

■ References

1. Why Doctors Can't Manage Money, Zena Kumok, Investopedia http://www.investopedia.com/articles/investing Accessed July 13 2015
2. Ibid
3. Parkinson CN. Parkinson's Law. Buccaneer Books;1996
4. Brokaw T. The Greatest Generation. New York, NY: Random House;2001

29 The Doctor's Day in Court

The practice of medicine and surgery has become more than the day-to-day practice of good medicine and surgery. Lawyers and regulators are hovering, waiting to pounce upon any opportunity to profit from any breakdown in the doctor-patient relationship.

"Third-party" predators can be government agencies, health insurance companies, members of the legal profession, ex-spouses, and former practice associates. So, how does a physician minimize the possibility of becoming the target of a legal action? The answer: to make it one's mission to understand the legal system and use every available resource to defend oneself against it. The following are points extracted from a presentation I frequently give at continuing education conventions and seminars to colleagues.

"The first thing you have to do to win is to keep from losing." So said one of the winningest coaches in college football history, Coach Paul "Bear" Bryant. The coach's secret to success applies in the medical profession, as well. So, how does a physician/surgeon "keep from losing"? The answer is by preparing for the day they might have to defend themself in a court of law or before a panel investigating accusations of wrongdoing.

The truth is that in the 21st century, there is a good chance that doctors have been—or will be—sued at some point in their career. You do not have to do something "wrong" to find yourself as a defendant in a malpractice suit; however, if/when you find yourself in the position of a defendant, it should be viewed as *an act of war*. You are fighting for your reputation. Take no prisoners. You are expected to fight fairly, but enter the arena with one though in mind: *to win!*

Immediately notify your malpractice insurance carrier that you either have received notice of a lawsuit, or may be expecting notification.

The plaintiff (usually a former patient) will be represented by an attorney. That attorney will hire an "expert witness" (usually a doctor in the same field of medicine/surgery as you). The plaintiff's expert's task it is to destroy your credibility. If that expert has been hired, you can bet they are prepared to testify—under oath—that you have committed "malpractice"; otherwise, the case will not get to trial.

The emotional response to being dragged into a lawsuit is one of dismay. The prudent response is to accept it as the price you pay for being a doctor, and prepare for your day in court.

Leading up to that day, your role is to teach your own attorney about the medicine/surgery of the case and become your own best advocate.

If you have done the things you should have done—as the president/CEO of your practice—the medical record will have been prepared for this day. From the first time the patient/plaintiff called your office to the last, every encounter, every conversation, every element of the treatment you provided will be accurately and legibly recorded in the patient's medical record.

Upon receiving notice of a suit, you should carefully study the *entire* record of the patient/plaintiff. If you discover a glaring error in the record and wish to "amend" it, make the correction in the margin or underneath the entry and write the word *Addendum* first; then enter the correction. Initial and date the entry. **Never, ever,** *alter* the medical record. Never erase or deface a previous entry. In the eyes of a jury, doing so amounts to an admission of guilt. Juries have been known to impose massive monetary judgments against doctors who attempted to alter the record or cover up evidence.

If you have contacted your malpractice carrier, you will have been told to make a complete and accurate copy of the medical record and file the copy in a safe place, away from the usual medical record storage site or location. Identify the copy—in bold print—**"IN ANTICIPATION OF LEGAL ACTION."** Keep all correspondence between you and your attorney and any notes you make about the case in the "anticipation" file. There, they are protected from "discovery" by the plaintiff's attorney. Do not discuss or release any information about the case to anyone other than your attorney or malpractice carrier.

At some point, you will be asked to give a "deposition." It will take place prior to your day in court, perhaps in your office or that of your attorney. Prepare for the deposition as you would for a board-certification examination. Review the patient's medical record and any hospital/surgicenter records that may apply. Commit them to memory, or at least know exactly where (in the record) the information about which you may be questioned can be retrieved during your deposition.

The purpose of most depositions is for the plaintiff's attorney to educate themself about the case.

A deposition begins in the same manner as a trial. You will be "sworn in," that is, asked to raise your right hand and swear to "tell the truth, the whole truth, and nothing but the truth." At all times, you must adhere to this oath, regardless of how painful it may be. On the other hand, your attorney will have already told you to answer the questions truthfully, but not to *volunteer* information. A brilliant attorney (Thomas Rhodes, Atlanta, Georgia) once told me, "You cannot win the case in a deposition, but you sure can lose it."

When answering a question, it is a good practice to say, "According to the record… " or "I noted in the patient's record that…" This gives your testimony credibility. And keep in mind that a court reporter is documenting every word you say. Your words are likely to be read aloud to you when you are on the witness stand at the time of trial. The plaintiff's attorney will attempt to cause you to contradict yourself, so pause and think before answering any—and every—question posed.

After the plaintiff's attorney has asked their questions, your attorney will have an opportunity to ask some and allow you to clarify anything you wish to clarify; but confer with your attorney (in private) if you need to.

It is also important to note that—*at any time*—during a deposition, if you should feel the need to confer with your attorney, simply say, "I'd like to take a break." You must be granted that request.

The plaintiff may attend your deposition. You should *absolutely* attend the deposition of the plaintiff. Sit across the table from the plaintiff and look into their eyes as they answer questions. You should also attend the deposition of the plaintiff's "expert" witness. If you feel that your attorney should follow up with a question or ask one that has not been asked, pass a note to your attorney. In short, participate in the process, *in a professional manner*. No one is more interested in your receiving justice than you are.

At some point the court reporter will provide your attorney with a full transcript of all depositions. Your attorney will make them available to you. Read every deposition relating to the case. Discuss your ideas with your attorney so that additional information can come out at trial.

It usually takes 3 to 4 years from the time you receive notification that a lawsuit has been filed before it goes to trial. So, you'll have plenty of time to prepare.

That will give you time to review all records obtained by your attorney, including all doctors, nurse practitioners, physician's assistants, dentists, rehabilitation specialists, and pharmacies that ever provided care for the patient/plaintiff. Go through the files to see if their records contain anything that could help you defend yourself, such as any pattern of noncompliance, drug addiction, or felonies.

When the date for court is set, cancel out an entire week from your office. Devote your undivided attention to winning the case. Before and after court, you'll meet with your attorney to discuss the upcoming events of the day or those passed and plan for the following day.

When you arrive at court, you should have left all jewelry (except a wedding band and understated watch) at home. Wear nonflashy clothes and accessories. Keep in mind the jury will size you up rather quickly. The more "like them" you are, the more apt they are to identify with you and the situation you are in.

Portray the image of a caring, considerate professional. Stand when the judge enters the room *and* when the jury enters and exits the room. Make eye contact with jurors, if possible. But make no gestures.

As in the deposition, the plaintiff gets to present evidence first. The first couple of days will be difficult for you. You will hear lies told about you and the care you and your staff provided bent in ways that you will hardly recognize it. Do not react in a manner that is distracting to the jury. There is nothing wrong with a slight shake of the head from side to side when a lie is told about you from the witness stand.

It is also appropriate for you to take notes during the trial. If you feel that your attorney should be following up on testimony given by other witnesses from the stand or the opposing legal team, pass your attorney a note. But be professional in your demeanor and mannerisms.

Once the plaintiff "rests," that is, completes putting on their case, your team will have the chance to do so. Your attorney will have secured an "expert witness" (colleague in the same field of medicine/surgery) who will testify that you *did not* commit malpractice. There may also be other witnesses to support your case.

Toward the end of the case, you will have "your day in court." You will go to the witness stand, swear to tell the truth, and answer questions from your attorney. This series of questions will be rather easy. You and your attorney will have rehearsed them. Your attorney already knows how you will answer the questions. This is your time to shine—to teach the jury about the medicine and/or surgery of the case. You may use props, photographs, drawing pads, or models to make your point. When you are asked questions (regardless of who asks them), turn to the jury and look each one of them in the eye as you answer. There is one exception. If the judge asks you a question, turn to the judge and begin your answer with "Your honor." Look the judge in the eye as you answer.

The plaintiff's attorney will also have a chance to question you while you are on the stand. Their objective is to trip you up and make you appear uncredible to the jury. Be respectful as you answer. Call the attorney by their last name, for example, "Mr. Smith, my best recollection is… " And keep in mind that the plaintiff's attorney likely asked you the same question in a slightly different way during your deposition.

In each case, pause after the question is asked, contemplate your answer, and then answer it as briefly as you can. If you can answer with a "Yes" or "No," do so. And do not allow the plaintiff's attorney to rattle you or put words in your mouth. Do not hesitate to say, "No, Mr. Smith, that is not correct… "

Your attorney will have another opportunity to question you while you are on the witness stand to help clear up any ambiguous points or elaborate on answers that will help your cause.

When all evidence has been presented, the judge will "charge" the jury, meaning the judge will inform them of the law and how they are expected to arrive at a decision. The jury will be excused and go to a private room to deliberate. They will examine all written and spoken evidence and render a verdict *for you* or *for the plaintiff*. It may take hours for them to agree, perhaps a day or so.

It is somewhat comforting to know that for the verdict to be decided in favor of the plaintiff (and against you), the jury's decision must be unanimous, that is, *every juror* must decide against you. History is on the side of the physician. The vast majority of cases are decided in the doctor's favor, unless gross negligence or wrongdoing has been committed, as is rarely the case.

The bottom line is the more you know about the legal system, the better you prepare every medical record for the possibility that it may become your best piece of evidence if—and when—you are sued, and the better prepared you are when you are deposed or when you go to court, the more apt you are to have the jury decide in your favor.

If you are known in your community as a physician who will be difficult to get a verdict returned against, the more likely the legal profession is to think twice before taking on a case against you.

Please be advised that the foregoing are my general thoughts and are not intended to be construed as legal advice. You should consult with your malpractice carrier representative and attorney and follow their advice.

30 The Way Forward

The final thoughts I share with future generations include the advice once given to me by my mentor Dr. Jack Anderson: *"as soon as possible get independent of hospitals and third-party payers."* Create an environment in which all contracts and agreements are between the patient and yourself.

Regarding your part of the contract, keep in mind that the vast majority of patients who consult a facial surgeon are not interested in a total transformation in their appearance. They simply want to look better, more rested, more youthful. It is a lesson too frequently learned through the treacherous method known as "trial and error." That will not be the case with readers of this book. You have a jump start on your colleagues, and competitors in other specialties who offer aesthetic and reconstructive procedures.

Never lose sight of a simple fact: *while a small percentage of the population want drastic changes in their appearance, most patients want to look "like themselves" (only younger), regardless of the products and techniques used.* And your task is to help them reach that goal.

It is the responsibility of the facial surgeon to be familiar with available options and to recommend a *condition-specific* combination of treatment modalities to each patient. Doing so separates artisans from technicians, thinkers and visionaries from mindless followers, askers of *why* from those who merely ask *how, what,* and *when.* Each generation of facial surgeons must resist the temptation to veer from the fundamental tenets that underlie its foundation—the *surgically oriented* foundation laid by its founding fathers.

The age-old idiom "Jack of all trades, master of none" also apples to physicians who specialize in facial surgery. A surgeon who attempts to be "all things to all people" loses the argument that they are *the source of surgical excellence in the head and neck.*

When facial surgeons fall into the trap of competing with nonsurgical specialties that can only offer nonsurgical procedures, we weaken our brand. And any Madison Avenue firm will tell you that when public perception about the unique niche of one's brand comes into question, the beginning of the end is within sight.

So, what is the answer to establishing an elite facial surgery practice that provides patients with a wide variety of procedures and products? In my opinion, the answer is to develop working relationships with health care providers qualified to provide procedures outside the head and neck region. Help them build their *nonfacial* surgery practices—to be so busy doing body and breast procedures, they won't have time to perform facial procedures.

A corollary to the above is to *also* develop relationships with health care providers who specialize in nonsurgical procedures. Assist them in building their *nonsurgical* practice in return for their assisting you in building your *surgical practice.* In this scenario, everybody wins—the surgeon, the nonsurgeon, and the patient. And what could be a better outcome than that? What better way is there to preserve the specialty's legacy?

Index